Touch Me with Love

Intimate Alignment for Couples Through Touch and Yoga

Touch Me with Love

Intimate Alignment for Couples Through Touch and Yoga

Touch Me with Love

Copyright © 2025 by Versandra Kennebrew
All rights reserved.

No part of this publication may be reproduced, stored in a retrieval system, or transmitted in any form or by any means—electronic, mechanical, photocopying, recording, or otherwise—without prior written permission from the publisher, except for brief quotations in critical reviews or articles.

Imprint:
Syntax Solutions L.C.
Columbus, Ga

Book Formatting Assistance & Design by:
Syntax Solutions L.C.

Photography by:
DSouyle

ISBN: 979-8-9878909-7-4

Cover Design by: Sun Rhythms

Printed in the United States of America

For permission, inquiries, or bulk orders, please contact:
www.versandrakennebrew.com

Intimate Alignment for Couples Through Touch and Yoga

Disclaimer

The content in this book is not intended to diagnose, treat, prevent or cure any disease or condition. It is not intended to be a substitute for the advice, treatment and/or diagnosis of a qualified licensed professional. It makes no medical diagnoses, claims or substitute for your personal physician's care.

As your holistic health coach, I do not provide a second opinion or in any way attempt to alter the treatment plans, therapeutic goals or recommendations of your personal physician. My role is to partner with you to provide ongoing support and accountability as you create an action plan to meet and maintain your health goals.

~Versandra Kennebrew, INHC

No part of this book may be reproduced or transmitted in any form or by any means electronic or mechanical, including photocopying, facsimile, recording, or by any information storage and retrieval system, without written permission from the author and/or publisher.

Syntax Solutions L.C. provided formatting, publishing, and/or design support for this book but is not responsible for the content, claims, or accuracy of the material presented. The views expressed are solely those of the author. Syntax Solutions L.C. assumes no liability for any outcomes, direct or indirect, resulting from the application or interpretation of this content.

Table Of Contents

AN URGENT CALL TO ACTION	V
FOREWORD	VI
PREFACE	IX
CHAPTER 1: INTRODUCTION TO INTIMATE ALIGNMENT	1
CHAPTER 2: UNDERSTANDING TOUCH	4
CHAPTER 3: THE FUNDAMENTALS OF YOGA	8
CHAPTER 4: CREATING A SHARED SPACE	11
CHAPTER 5: BREATH AND TOUCH	14
CHAPTER 6: PARTNER YOGA TECHNIQUES	17
CHAPTER 7: TOUCH TECHNIQUES FOR HEALING	20
CHAPTER 8: BUILDING EMOTIONAL INTIMACY	23
CHAPTER 9: NAVIGATING CHALLENGES TOGETHER	26
CHAPTER 10: CULTIVATING A DAILY PRACTICE	29
CHAPTER 11: CELEBRATING YOUR JOURNEY	32
CHAPTER 12: RESOURCES AND FURTHER READING	35

CHAPTER 13: WELCOME TO THE ART OF TOUCH EXPERIENCE	41
CHAPTER 14: MISCONCEPTIONS ABOUT TOUCH	47
CHAPTER 15: APPROPRIATE & INAPPROPRIATE TOUCH	50
CHAPTER 16: TOUCH TRAUMA	54
CHAPTER 17: YOU FEEL ME?	58
CHAPTER 18: CONCLUSION	60
ABOUT THE AUTHOR	63

AN URGENT CALL TO ACTION

Dr. Vivek Murthy, a former U.S. Surgeon General, has identified loneliness and isolation as a significant public health crisis in the United States. In his recent advisory, "Our Epidemic of Loneliness and Isolation: The Surgeon General's Advisory on the Healing Effects of Social Connection and Community," he highlights the crucial role of meaningful connections in enhancing individual and community health, safety, prosperity, and overall well-being.

The advisory points out the public health risks associated with loneliness and social disconnection, referencing studies that show around half of U.S. adults report experiencing notable levels of loneliness. The absence of social connections can lead to severe health issues, including a higher likelihood of coronary heart disease, stroke, diabetes, depression, anxiety, and early death. Couples reading this book will have a unique opportunity to help themselves while supporting their entire family during this public health crisis.

FOREWORD

As human beings, our brains are hard-wired to experience connection. Regardless of a person's age, gender, ethnicity, financial status, etc., we all have a need to love and to be loved. This is something that is formulated within us before we are even born. While we are in the process of gestation in our mother's womb, we can hear and feel her heartbeat. We quite literally grow and develop inside of another human being, relying totally on our mother's bodies to keep us alive. If you are reading these words, it is because you were successfully kept safe within your mother's womb for the first several months of your body's existence.

Once we are finally born, we then sup from our mother's bosom, being fed a substance produced from her body that continues to sustain us. During the moments of breastfeeding, oxytocin, the bonding hormone that creates a sense of connection, is released within our mother and within us. This is true for virtually all mammals but none more significantly than in humans. It is part of the design by which we were created, and it is a good design.

Connection is a beautiful thing, and it is so vital to our sense of wellbeing that we do all sorts of things in an effort to experience it. While there are certainly some unhealthy approaches that people take to experience connection, appropriate, loving physical touch can be a highly beneficial way we can have this primal need fulfilled. It can at once create an experience of connection as well as healing. The Bible even mentions healing taking place through the laying on of hands.

When I think about the healing power of touch and when I think of a person touching someone with love, I think of Versandra Kennebrew. Many years ago, in a building with many business offices, I saw on the marquee a business called "The Healing Power of Touch." I was immediately intrigued and made my way to that office to see what it was about. Immediately upon entering, I could tell that it was a healing space. I met several kindhearted massage therapists who worked there, including Versandra, the proprietor of the business who, at that time, was a relatively recent graduate of the acclaimed Irene's Myomassology Institute. From ongoing conversations with Versandra, the depth of her training and knowledge were clear. Moreover, her passion for people and commitment to being a force for good and a vessel of healing consistently showed on full display.

There was one unforgettable experience that took place a few months after meeting Versandra in 2002 that illustrates that perfectly. Although she and I had different areas of expertise as vessels of healing, we have always respected one another's gifts and proficiencies. In that context, Versandra shared with me about a person who was having some significant health challenges. She appeared to be in the process of making her transition. Versandra was going to offer this lady a massage, although there was going to be no payment for her services, and she asked if I would be willing to go with her to offer healing support via the modality that I utilize. I agreed to do so.

We arrived at a home where a lady answered the door. We entered the home, and inside was her mother. She was completely incapacitated, unconscious, and unresponsive. I watched Versandra massage this unconscious woman in a way, unlike anything I had ever seen before. The love with which she touched this lady, whom, to the best of my knowledge, she didn't even know, was awe-inspiring. That was well over 20 years ago, but it impacted me so significantly that I have never forgotten it and doubt that I ever will. With each touch, each intentional stroke upon this woman's skin, I could see exuding through Versandra's hands an outpouring of love so graceful, warm, and kind that I couldn't help but be astonished as I observed. In Versandra's face, I could see the intention of love and peace that she was endeavoring to pour into this lady.

Everything about her entire being said, "If there's anything I can do to have a positive impact on this lady's well-being, I'm going to pour everything good into her that I possibly can."

I never saw that lady again after that day. I don't know how much longer she lived after that, whether a day, a week, or a year, but I know that before she left this planet, she had a lot of love poured into her. I also know that Versandra had a lot of love pouring through her that day, and I am sure many days since then.

There is something truly beautiful and even reciprocal that takes place when one offers another the opportunity to experience the healing power of touch by touching that person with love. Yet, that's the nature of how life unfolds. That which we intend towards others also makes its way back to us, and the heart space we operate from in our intentions and actions impact not only the recipient of whom our actions are intended towards, but us as well. It has a soul level impact even if we're not consciously aware of it.

But there are things that we can do consciously and intentionally, and that is to resolve that we are going to show up as beacons of love. Do you choose to show up as a beacon of love? Do you aim to be a force for good? Is the idea of touching your beloved in such a way that you both get to experience a deeper level of connection, love, and harmony appealing to you? If your answer is yes to any or all of these questions, then you are in the right place. In this book, "Touch Me with Love," Versandra will masterfully take you on a journey that will awaken you to a new level of awareness, more fully activate your heart center, and empower you to take your love life to a new level. EnJOY.

Rev. Royce Fletcher Thomason, Developer of Transcending the Matrix Healing System

PREFACE

Grandma Nina Bell would say, "Come here baby and scratch grandma's scalp." There were six decades between us, and her persona was strong and hard. Because my grandma was born in a time when corporal punishment was commonplace, she demonstrated her love with switches, belts, or an unexpected backhand from time to time.

Her softer side was expressed during our grooming time together. Besides gentle scratching with the big tooth comb on her scalp, she also enjoyed me scrubbing her back with the big hand towel (or so it seemed with my little hands) while in the bath. But it was the memory of rubbing grandma's specially concocted liniment on her shoulders, back and knees to help relieve her pain that inspired me to become a myomassologist as a second career.

The journey of a massage practitioner is intense to say the least. With no prior college education and having only read about massage and seen pictures in magazines, I was ignorant about what I was getting into. There I was, on the cusp of becoming forty years of age, and I was feeling this intense pull toward an ancient healing practice that required me to study anatomy, physiology, pathology and an array of other holistic practices. Simultaneously, my spiritual world was being shaken to the core. God was being revealed to me on a level I didn't believe was possible.

As I touched more people and truly connected to their pain, their joy, and their losses, my capacity to love without judgement was expanded. I learned to see God, the all-encompassing everywhere evenly present force that binds everything that is in everyone and everything, everywhere. Studying the healing arts and being aware of the power of God moving through me in support of another changed my life. The oneness of God became crystal clear.

Don't get me wrong, this new awareness was not appreciated by those closest to me. My father would not allow me to give him a massage because in his words, "you're my daughter, you can't give me a massage." Other members of my family believed I was losing it. You see, twenty-five years ago, holistic health practitioners were not understood or valued in the mainstream. It appeared that the rich, famous, and eclectic were indulging in these complementary and alternative medicine practices and everyday people were just trying to see what was behind the veil. My dad introduced me as his eclectic daughter.

At the same time, the World Health Organization (WHO) and *institutions* like the University of Florida were conducting research that would unveil to North America knowledge that had been understood in the East for millennia. This groundwork was establishing a presence for medical and sports massage therapy in television, films, and healthcare facilities.

My portable massage chair and table have traveled with me throughout the U.S. and Canada. I've had the privilege of working with Kirk Whalum, my favorite saxophonist, Lin Rountree, the jazz funk trumpeter, "The Motivator" Les Brown, esteemed artists, and even political figures who sought my services. I provided massage therapy to the wealthy and well-known, and my team and I catered to corporate clients such as Ford Motor Company, Blue Cross Blue Shield, among many others.

After completing three thousand massage sessions, I stopped keeping track, but feedback from workshop participants indicated that my specialty lies in teaching the art of touch. While my goal was to create a system for couples to connect through non-verbal communication via touch, attendees emphasized that self-massage for self-care should also be a key focus.

Looking back twenty years, I see that God was speaking to practitioners and laypeople alike concerning the need for human connection. Cuddle parties started popping up as a solution to the need for connection and intimacy. Australian man Juan Mann started the Free Hugs Campaign to remedy his personal feelings of loneliness and sadness, and like wildfire, this social movement spread around the world. People were using social media and popular news outlets to galvanize those who wanted to spread love and hope to strangers in public places.

I had finally discovered my happy place. Studying yoga at the Kashi Atlanta Urban Ashram provided me with what I felt was the missing piece of the puzzle. The newfound understanding of the power of breath, mindfulness, and synchronistic movement enriched the Art of Touch Experiences and Retreats. I overcame my fears and embraced oneness with nature. Hosting retreats in stunning state parks and outdoor locations, along with virtual in-home retreats, opened up more opportunities for sharing the art of touch and supporting couples globally.

The need for intimate alignment within our communities is more evident today than ever before. Former United States Surgeon General Vivek Murthy, an American physician who served as the 19th and 21st Surgeon General, made significant contributions during his eight-year tenure. He underscored the critical point that the most pressing public health crisis of our time is not just loneliness, but also a profound lack of meaningful connection among individuals.

We have got to reconnect as a society, and it is my heartfelt desire to live out my days teaching newlyweds and couples the essential skills needed to achieve true intimacy alignment. Couples will then pass on this invaluable knowledge to their children, and in turn, those children will teach their own children the vital lesson that we need one another to thrive and survive in this world.

Note to reader: This is not a read it and put it on a shelf book. Whether you are reading the flipbook, eBook, or hard copy of the manuscript, plan to reference the words and multimedia content often and maybe even with a companion. Enjoy your co-creations.

CHAPTER 1: INTRODUCTION TO INTIMATE ALIGNMENT

The Power of Touch in Relationships

The power of touch in relationships is a profound aspect that extends beyond mere physical interaction. It plays a crucial role in fostering intimacy and connection between partners. Touch can communicate feelings that words sometimes fail to express, creating an emotional bond that enhances the relationship. For couples and newlyweds, understanding the significance of touch can deepen their connection, promoting a healthy and nurturing environment conducive to growth and love.

When couples engage in touch, whether through holding hands, hugging, or gentle caresses, they trigger the release of oxytocin, often referred to as the "love hormone." This hormone is essential in building trust and emotional closeness. The act of touching can reduce stress and anxiety levels, leading to a more harmonious relationship. As couples incorporate touch into their daily routines, they establish a sense of security and safety, which is vital for open communication and vulnerability.

Yoga offers an excellent platform to integrate touch into relationships. Partner yoga practices encourage physical closeness and mutual support, allowing couples to experience the benefits of touch in a mindful way. Through synchronized movements and shared postures, partners can enhance their awareness of each other's bodies, promoting a sense of unity. This shared experience not only strengthens their physical connection but also deepens their emotional ties, allowing them to communicate non-verbally through their movements and presence.

Moreover, the practice of mindful touch during yoga can help couples develop a deeper understanding of each other's needs and boundaries. Engaging in gentle, intentional touch fosters a greater awareness of feelings and sensations, encouraging couples to be more attuned to each other. This awareness is essential in navigating the complexities of relationships, as it cultivates empathy and compassion. As partners learn to communicate through touch, they create a safe space where both individuals feel valued and understood.

Ultimately, the power of touch in relationships cannot be underestimated. For couples and newlyweds, integrating touch through practices like yoga can significantly enhance their emotional and physical connection. By prioritizing touch, partners can foster a loving and supportive environment that nurtures their relationship. Embracing the transformative potential of touch not only strengthens bonds but also promotes overall well-being, paving the way for a fulfilling and lasting partnership.

The Role of Yoga in Enhancing Connection

In the pursuit of deeper intimacy and connection, yoga emerges as a powerful tool for couples. The practice of yoga encourages couples to move together, breathe together, and exist in a shared space of mindfulness. This shared experience fosters a sense of unity and understanding, allowing partners to cultivate a more profound emotional and physical connection. As couples engage in yoga, they not only enhance their individual well-being but also strengthen the bond that ties them together.

One of the primary ways yoga enhances connection is through synchronized movements. When couples practice yoga side by side, they engage in a dance of harmony and support. Each pose requires a level of awareness and attention to one another, creating an environment where partners can communicate non-verbally. This physical synchronization helps couples learn to trust each other, as they rely on one another for balance and stability. The result is a deepened sense of partnership that extends beyond the yoga mat and into everyday life.

Another essential aspect of yoga is the emphasis on breath. In yoga, breath serves as a bridge between the mind and body, helping individuals to center themselves in the present moment. For couples, synchronized breathing can significantly enhance their emotional connection. When partners breathe together, they create a shared rhythm, which can lead to a greater sense of calm and understanding. This practice encourages couples to be more attuned to each other's emotional states, fostering empathy and compassion.

Mindfulness is a cornerstone of yoga that plays a crucial role in deepening intimacy. By practicing mindfulness together, couples can learn to cultivate awareness of each other's needs and feelings. This heightened awareness allows partners to respond to one another with greater sensitivity and care. Engaging in mindfulness practices during yoga not only strengthens the connection between partners but also enhances their ability to navigate challenges together. This shared journey towards mindfulness can lead to healthier communication patterns and a more resilient relationship.

Finally, incorporating touch into yoga practice deepens the connection couples share. Touch is an essential human need, and in yoga, it can manifest through partner poses, gentle adjustments, or simple handholding during meditation. These moments of physical contact reinforce feelings of safety and security, further solidifying the bond between partners. By integrating touch with yoga, couples create a sacred space where vulnerability is welcomed, allowing for a greater exploration of intimacy and connection. As partners continue to practice together, they build a foundation of trust and affection that can enrich their relationship for years to come.

CHAPTER 2: UNDERSTANDING TOUCH

The Science of Touch

The Science of Touch delves into the profound effects that tactile interactions have on human relationships, particularly for couples. Touch is not merely a physical act; it is a complex interplay between physiological, psychological, and emotional elements. Research shows that tactile stimulation can release oxytocin, often referred to as the "love hormone," which fosters bonding and intimacy. This biochemical response underscores the importance of touch in nurturing relationships and enhancing feelings of trust and security between partners. For newlyweds, establishing a strong foundation of physical affection can significantly enrich their emotional connection and overall relationship satisfaction.

Incorporating touch into daily routines can also have beneficial health effects. Studies indicate that regular physical contact can lower stress levels by reducing cortisol, the body's primary stress hormone. When couples engage in affectionate behaviors like hugging, holding hands, or gentle caresses, they experience not only emotional warmth but also physiological benefits. This reduction in stress enhances overall well-being, making it easier for couples to navigate the challenges of their new life together. By integrating touch into their yoga practice, couples can amplify these health benefits, combining the calming effects of yoga with the nurturing power of touch.

The benefits of touch also play a critical role in emotional regulation. Couples who regularly engage in affectionate touch report higher levels of happiness and satisfaction in their relationships. The act of touching serves as a non-verbal form of communication, conveying feelings that words sometimes cannot express. For newlyweds, developing a language of touch can be particularly beneficial as they navigate the early stages of marriage. By learning to read each other's signals and responding accordingly, couples can build a more resilient and harmonious partnership.

Ultimately, the science of touch emphasizes the importance of physical connection in fostering intimacy and health for couples. As newlyweds embark on their journey together, integrating touch into their shared experiences, including their yoga practice, can create a lasting bond that enhances their relationship. By understanding the physiological and emotional impacts of touch, couples can cultivate an environment ripe for love, understanding, and growth. This approach not only enhances their individual well-being but also solidifies the foundation for a thriving partnership.

Types of Touch and Their Benefits

Touch is a fundamental form of communication that extends beyond words, playing a vital role in human connection, especially in intimate relationships. Understanding the various types of touch can enhance the bond between couples, fostering deeper emotional and physical intimacy. The different forms of touch include affectionate touch, supportive touch, playful touch, sensual touch, and healing touch, each serving unique purposes and offering distinct benefits.

Affectionate touch, such as hugging, holding hands, or cuddling, promotes feelings of safety and belonging. For newlyweds, adding frequent doses of affectionate touch into daily routines can enhance relationship satisfaction and reinforce feelings of love and appreciation. Simple gestures like a warm embrace can be powerful in maintaining a strong emotional bond.

Supportive touch often comes in the form of a reassuring pat on the back or a gentle squeeze of the hand during challenging times. This type of touch communicates empathy and understanding, providing comfort and reassurance when needed most. Couples can benefit from integrating supportive touch not only during moments of stress but also as a proactive approach to nurturing their relationship. By consistently offering supportive touches, partners can foster an environment of trust and emotional safety.

Playful touch, such as tickling or playful nudges, introduces an element of fun and spontaneity into the relationship. Engaging in playful touch can lighten the mood and create shared joyful experiences that strengthen the connection between partners. This type of interaction encourages laughter and fosters a sense of partnership, allowing couples to navigate challenges together with a lighter heart. Incorporating playful touch into daily life can enhance overall relationship satisfaction and help couples stay connected through shared enjoyment.

Sensual touch focuses on physical intimacy, enhancing the romantic aspect of a relationship. This can include gentle caresses, massages, or other forms of intimate contact that deepen physical attraction. Sensual touch is essential for maintaining a vibrant sexual connection, which is crucial for many couples. It encourages vulnerability and openness, allowing partners to explore their desires and strengthen their bond. Practicing sensual touch alongside yoga can also enhance body awareness, making the experience more fulfilling and connected.

Healing touch encompasses therapeutic forms of touch, such as massage or gentle bodywork, aimed at alleviating stress and promoting relaxation. This type of touch can be especially beneficial for couples looking to integrate health and wellness practices into their relationship. By prioritizing healing touch, partners can support each other's physical and emotional well-being, creating a nurturing environment that encourages growth and healing. Combining healing touch with yoga practices can enhance relaxation and mindfulness, further deepening the intimate alignment between partners.

CHAPTER 3: THE FUNDAMENTALS OF YOGA

Yoga Philosophy for Couples

Yoga philosophy offers valuable insights for couples seeking deeper connections and harmonious relationships. At its core, yoga teaches the importance of unity and balance, principles that are essential in a partnership. By understanding and applying these philosophical tenets, couples can create a nurturing environment that fosters intimacy, trust, and mutual growth. This subchapter will explore key aspects of yoga philosophy that can enhance the bonds between partners and encourage a shared journey of discovery and healing.

One of the foundational concepts in yoga philosophy is the idea of non-attachment, or "Aparigraha." In a romantic relationship, this principle encourages partners to cultivate love without clinging or possessiveness. By practicing non-attachment, couples can learn to appreciate each other's individuality while maintaining a sense of togetherness. This balance allows for personal growth and self-exploration, enabling each partner to flourish without fear of losing their identity. As couples embrace this philosophy, they can create a space where both partners feel safe to express themselves authentically.

Another essential element of yoga philosophy is the practice of mindfulness, which emphasizes awareness of the present moment. For couples, being mindful in their interactions can deepen their emotional connection. Mindfulness encourages partners to listen actively, respond thoughtfully, and engage fully in their shared experiences. By incorporating mindfulness into their daily routines, couples can transform ordinary moments into opportunities for intimacy, whether through shared yoga practices, deep conversations, or simply enjoying each other's company. This heightened awareness fosters a sense of appreciation and gratitude, reinforcing the bond between partners.

The concept of "Sankalpa," or intention-setting, plays a significant role in yoga philosophy as well. Couples can benefit from establishing shared intentions that align with their values and aspirations. By collaboratively defining their goals and dreams, partners can create a roadmap for their relationship, guiding them through challenges and celebrations alike. This practice of setting intentions not only enhances communication but also strengthens the commitment between partners, as they work together towards a common vision. In this way, Sankalpa serves as a powerful tool for cultivating a resilient and fulfilling partnership.

Lastly, the principle of "Ahimsa," or non-violence, is fundamental to yoga philosophy and has profound implications for couples. This principle encourages compassion and understanding in all interactions, promoting a safe and supportive environment for both partners. By practicing Ahimsa, couples can navigate conflicts with kindness and respect, recognizing that disagreements are a natural part of any relationship. This approach fosters emotional safety and creates a foundation of trust, allowing couples to grow together while facing life's challenges. As partners embrace these philosophical teachings, they can cultivate a relationship that is not only loving but also deeply aligned with their shared values and aspirations.

Essential Yoga Poses for Connection

Yoga offers a profound way for couples to connect with each other on both physical and emotional levels. By practicing specific poses together, couples can enhance their intimacy and deepen their bond. These poses not only promote physical alignment and relaxation but also encourage communication and trust. As you embark on this journey of connection, consider incorporating the following essential yoga poses into your practice.

One of the foundational poses for couples is a variation of the partner tree pose. In this pose, one partner stands tall and props the heal of their right foot against their left inner ankle while the other leans against them, creating a shared sense of stability. The standing partner grounds themselves by finding their center, while the other can focus on balancing with their left foot on their tight ankle and leaning into their partner for support. This pose symbolizes mutual trust and reliance, fostering a sense of security in the relationship. Practicing this pose regularly can help couples develop a deeper understanding of each other's strengths and vulnerabilities.

Another effective pose is the seated forward fold, where couples sit facing each other, legs extended and their feet touching. Partners can hold hands or for more support hold on to one another's wrists. As one partner leans forward, the other gently pulls them into a stretch and vice versa, creating a dynamic of give-and-take. This pose encourages open communication, allowing partners to express their needs and desires. The physical closeness enhances emotional intimacy, as couples can engage in eye contact and synchronized breathing. This shared experience not only releases physical tension but also nurtures a supportive space for vulnerability.

The double downward dog pose is a playful yet powerful way for couples to connect. In this pose, one partner assumes the downward dog position while the other places their hands on their partner's back, creating a supportive bridge. This interaction fosters a sense of teamwork and collaboration, as both partners work together to maintain balance and alignment. The physical touch involved in this pose can be invigorating, enhancing the couple's sense of connection and reinforcing the notion that they are stronger together.

A final essential pose is the heart-to-heart pose, where partners sit back-to-back, aligning their spines while maintaining a sense of openness. This position encourages couples to share their energy while also allowing for individual reflection. As partners sit in silence, they can focus on their breathing and the sensations in their bodies. This mindful practice cultivates a deeper awareness of each other's presence and encourages emotional vulnerability. Regularly practicing this pose can help couples foster a deeper connection and appreciation for their partner's emotional landscape.

Incorporating these essential yoga poses into your routine can significantly enhance the connection between partners. The combination of physical touch, shared experiences, and mindful communication creates a foundation for intimacy and trust. As couples engage in these poses together, they not only improve their physical health but also nurture their emotional bonds, paving the way for a fulfilling and harmonious relationship.

CHAPTER 4: CREATING A SHARED SPACE

Setting Up Your Yoga Area

Creating a dedicated yoga area at home can significantly enhance your practice as a couple, fostering intimacy and a shared commitment to wellness. Begin by selecting a space that is quiet and free from distractions. This could be a corner of your living room, a spare room, or even a section of your garden. The ideal space should allow for ample movement and be large enough to accommodate both partners comfortably. A serene environment is crucial, so consider how natural light, ventilation, and privacy can contribute to a calming atmosphere.

Next, focus on the flooring. A stable, non-slip surface is essential for practicing yoga safely. If your chosen area has hard flooring, consider using yoga mats or thick rugs to provide cushioning and traction. Ensure that both partners have their own mats, as this not only encourages individual practice but also emphasizes the importance of personal space within your shared journey. If you prefer a softer surface, a well-padded carpet can also work, as long as it allows for stable footing.

Now, think about the ambiance of your yoga space. Incorporating elements that evoke calmness, and tranquility will enhance your experience. Soft lighting, such as lamps or candles, can create a warm environment. You may also want to include plants or flowers, which can bring a touch of nature indoors and help purify the air. Consider adding calming scents through essential oils or incense, which can enhance relaxation and focus during your practice. Music can also play a role; select soothing tunes or nature sounds to create a peaceful soundscape.

Incorporate props and tools that can aid in your practice and encourage touch. Blocks, straps, and bolsters can enhance flexibility and support during poses, making your practice more enjoyable and effective. Additionally, having a soft blanket on hand can be useful for restorative poses or for cuddling together at the end of your session. These props encourage exploration and playfulness, which is essential for couples looking to deepen their connection through yoga.

Finally, establish a routine for maintaining your yoga area. Keeping the space tidy and organized can help reinforce the importance of your practice. Set aside time each week to clean and refresh your space, perhaps even involving a ritual that you both enjoy, like rearranging decorations or changing the scents you use. This not only keeps the area inviting but also reinforces the commitment you share to nurturing your relationship through touch and yoga. By creating a harmonious environment, you lay the foundation for a practice that is both intimate and enriching, enhancing your journey together.

Incorporating Touch into Your Environment

Creating a nurturing environment that incorporates touch can significantly enhance the emotional and physical well-being of couples, especially newlyweds. The space you inhabit should reflect a sense of intimacy and comfort, fostering connection and promoting shared experiences. Simple changes, such as rearranging furniture to encourage closeness or adding soft textiles, can create an inviting atmosphere conducive to touch. Consider using warm colors and gentle lighting to evoke a sense of relaxation and safety, making it easier for partners to engage in physical interaction.

Incorporating touch into your environment extends beyond aesthetics; it also involves creating opportunities for physical connection. Designate specific areas in your home for relaxation and intimacy, such as a cozy corner with cushions where you can sit close together or a yoga space that invites shared practice. This intentional arrangement encourages you to engage in activities that promote touch, such as partner yoga or guided relaxation exercises. By establishing these spaces, you not only foster a sense of intimacy but also communicate the importance of physical connection in your relationship.

The sensory elements of your environment also play a crucial role in enhancing the experience of touch. Introduce materials that feel good to the skin, such as soft blankets, plush pillows, and smooth stones. Aromatic scents can also heighten the experience of touch, as certain fragrances are known to promote relaxation and intimacy. Consider using essential oils or scented candles to create a calming atmosphere during your shared yoga practice or intimate moments. Engaging multiple senses can deepen your connection and make the experience of touch more profound and enjoyable.

In addition to physical modifications, communication is essential in incorporating touch into your environment. Discuss with your partner what types of touch feel most comforting and intimate to each of you. This dialogue encourages mutual understanding and respect for each other's boundaries and preferences. You might find that simple gestures, such as holding hands or cuddling while watching a movie, create a deeper sense of connection. Establishing a routine that includes touch can also enhance your bond, making it a natural part of your daily interactions.

Ultimately, incorporating touch into your environment is about creating a sanctuary for intimacy and connection. As you embark on this journey together, be mindful of the ways you can enhance your shared space to encourage physical closeness.

Whether through intentional design, sensory experiences, or open communication, nurturing a touch-friendly environment can significantly enrich your relationship. By prioritizing touch, you are not only promoting health and well-being but also cultivating a deeper emotional bond that will serve as a foundation for your life together.

CHAPTER 5: BREATH AND TOUCH

The Connection Between Breath and Touch

In the realm of intimate relationships, breath and touch serve as fundamental components of connection and communication. Understanding how these two elements interplay can enhance the bond between couples, particularly in the context of yoga and holistic health. Breath is often referred to as the life force, a vital energy that sustains our being. When combined with touch, it creates a powerful synergy that fosters deeper intimacy and understanding between partners. By learning to synchronize breath with touch, couples can cultivate a heightened sense of awareness and presence, enhancing their overall relationship.

Breath serves as a bridge between the mind and body, allowing individuals to access their emotional states and physical sensations. In moments of touch, whether through gentle caresses or more intentional therapeutic practices, the breath can guide the experience. For instance, during a shared yoga session, partners can focus on their breath as they move together, aligning their physical movements with their inhalations and exhalations. This integration not only deepens physical connection but also promotes emotional resonance, as partners become attuned to each other's rhythms and needs.

Touch, in contrast, is an immediate and visceral experience that conveys affection, comfort, and safety. The skin is rich with sensory receptors, making touch a profound way to communicate love and support. Couples can enhance their connection by consciously incorporating touch into their shared practices. Simple gestures like holding hands, hugging, or massaging each other can be enriched by mindful breathing. For example, when one partner breathes deeply while the other applies gentle pressure, it can create a sense of grounding and relaxation that strengthens their bond.

The combination of breath and touch can also facilitate healing on multiple levels. In yoga, various postures can encourage the release of tension and stress, while conscious breathing promotes emotional release and clarity. When partners engage in these practices together, they nurture not only their physical bodies but also their emotional health. This shared journey can lead to deeper understanding and compassion, allowing couples to support each other through challenges and celebrate victories together. The healing power of this synergy can transform the dynamics of a relationship, fostering resilience and unity.

Ultimately, the connection between breath and touch is a pathway to greater intimacy for couples. By consciously integrating these practices into their daily lives, newlyweds can cultivate a nurturing environment that encourages exploration and growth. As they deepen their understanding of each other through breath and touch, they can create a foundation of trust and love that will sustain them throughout their journey together. In this way, breath and touch become not just practices, but essential tools for fostering a harmonious and fulfilling relationship.

Breathing Exercises for Couples

Breathing exercises for couples play a crucial role in enhancing intimacy and connection. When partners engage in synchronized breathing, they not only promote relaxation but also cultivate a profound sense of unity. This practice encourages couples to attune to each other's rhythms, creating a shared space where they can explore their emotional and physical connection. By focusing on breath, couples can deepen their bond and foster a safe environment for open communication.

To begin, couples can sit comfortably facing each other, ensuring that they are relaxed and free from distractions. One effective technique is the "Coherent Breathing" exercise, where both partners inhale deeply for a count of five and exhale for a count of five. This rhythm encourages harmony and can help relieve stress. As partners breathe together, they can hold each other's hands, allowing the physical touch to reinforce the emotional connection. This synchronization not only calms the nervous system but also enhances feelings of safety and trust.

Another valuable exercise is the "Breath of Fire," which involves rapid, rhythmic breathing through the nose. This energizing practice can invigorate both partners, helping to release tension and increase vitality. It is essential for each partner to maintain awareness of their individual experiences while remaining connected. As they breathe in this manner, they can exchange glances or smiles, reinforcing their bond and enhancing the overall experience. This exercise is particularly beneficial before engaging in deeper practices like yoga or massage, as it prepares the body and mind for intimacy.

Incorporating visualization into breathing exercises can further enhance the experience. Couples can imagine their breaths as waves, flowing in and out, carrying away stress and inviting in peace. This visualization can be accompanied by affirmations such as, "We are connected," or "We support each other." Such affirmations can deepen the emotional connection, allowing couples to express their feelings and intentions non-verbally. The act of visualizing together can create a shared mental space that strengthens their relationship and fosters a deeper understanding of each other's needs.

Finally, integrating breathing exercises into a daily routine can significantly impact a couple's relationship. Setting aside time to practice together not only enhances physical health but also nurtures emotional intimacy. As couples continue to explore these techniques, they can adapt them to fit their unique dynamics, ensuring that the practice remains meaningful and enjoyable. Over time, consistent engagement with breathing exercises can lead to a more profound sense of alignment, both physically and emotionally, enriching their journey together in intimacy and health.

CHAPTER 6: PARTNER YOGA TECHNIQUES

Introduction to Partner Yoga

Partner yoga, a practice designed for two, invites couples to explore the dynamic between physical alignment and emotional connection. This form of yoga emphasizes synchronized movements and shared breath, fostering a deeper sense of intimacy. As newlyweds navigate the early stages of their relationship, partner yoga offers a unique opportunity to cultivate trust and support through shared physical experiences. This practice not only enhances flexibility and strength but also encourages emotional bonding, making it an ideal addition to a couple's journey toward a harmonious life together.

In partner yoga, the essence of touch plays a pivotal role. The gentle, supportive contact between partners can enhance the overall experience, allowing them to connect beyond verbal communication. Touch has profound implications for emotional health, as it releases oxytocin, the hormone associated with bonding. By integrating touch into their yoga practice, couples can deepen their understanding of each other's physical and emotional needs. This connection becomes an essential tool for nurturing a strong, resilient relationship built on mutual respect and affection.

The physical postures in partner yoga often require cooperation and communication. As couples engage in various poses, they learn to listen to each other's bodies, adapting their movements to create a balanced flow. This practice not only strengthens the body but also enhances the couple's ability to work together harmoniously. Through shared effort, partners develop a greater appreciation for each other's strengths and vulnerabilities, fostering a sense of unity that can translate into other aspects of their relationship.

Moreover, partner yoga serves as a platform for couples to explore their boundaries in a safe and nurturing environment. As they engage in physical poses, they may encounter discomfort or challenges that require them to communicate openly. This vulnerability is crucial for fostering trust and understanding, allowing couples to navigate their relationship with greater ease. By embracing the challenges of partner yoga, couples can build resilience, learning to support each other through both physical and emotional trials.

Ultimately, partner yoga is not just a physical practice; it is a holistic approach to nurturing intimacy and connection. As couples embark on this journey, they will discover the profound benefits of integrating touch and movement into their relationship. The experience encourages couples to deepen their connection, enhancing not only their physical health but also their emotional well-being. Through the shared practice of partner yoga, newlyweds can lay a strong foundation for a loving, supportive partnership that thrives on intimacy and mutual growth.

Key Poses for Couples

In the journey of intimacy and connection, yoga offers a unique opportunity for couples to deepen their bond through shared physical practice. Key poses specifically designed for couples not only enhance physical alignment but also foster emotional closeness. These poses encourage communication, trust, and a sense of unity, making them ideal for newlyweds who are exploring their relationship's depths. Each pose serves as a tool to integrate touch and health, creating a shared experience that can strengthen both body and relationship.

One of the foundational poses for couples is the seated back-to-back position. In this pose, partners sit with their backs aligned, allowing them to connect and support each other's posture. This position emphasizes the importance of trust, as each partner leans into the other for balance. It encourages deep breathing, helping couples synchronize their breaths and creating a harmonious energy flow. This pose not only enhances physical alignment but also cultivates a deeper emotional connection, facilitating open communication and mutual support.

Another essential pose is the partner forward fold. In this pose, one partner stands behind the other, who is bending forward while holding onto their partner's wrists or forearms. This pose emphasizes the idea of support and surrender, as one partner provides a grounding presence, the other relaxes into the stretch. This act of touch and support enhances feelings of safety and connection, reinforcing the notion that partners can rely on each other during challenging moments. The forward fold also promotes flexibility and openness in both the body and the relationship.

The partner tree pose is another excellent way to cultivate balance and connection. In this pose, couples stand side by side, each lifting one leg to rest on the inner thigh or calf of the opposite leg. By holding hands, they create a mutual support system that enhances stability and alignment. This pose illustrates the beauty of interdependence, showing that while each partner has their individual strength, they can flourish together. Practicing the partner tree pose encourages couples to communicate their needs and find a shared balance, both physically and emotionally.

Incorporating these key poses into a couple's routine not only fosters physical fitness but also nurtures a deeper emotional connection. Through shared experiences on the mat, couples can explore their own vulnerabilities while building trust and understanding. As they navigate the challenges and joys of life together, these poses serve as reminders of their commitment to each other. By integrating touch for health with yoga, newlyweds can create a strong foundation for their relationship, paving the way for a lifetime of intimacy and growth.

CHAPTER 7: TOUCH TECHNIQUES FOR HEALING

Massage Techniques for Couples

Massage can be a profound way for couples to connect, deepen intimacy, and enhance overall well-being. Understanding various massage techniques can help partners create a nurturing environment that fosters relaxation and strengthens their bond. These techniques are not only beneficial for physical health but also serve as a means to communicate love and care through touch. By learning and practicing these methods together, couples can experience a shared journey toward greater harmony and alignment in their relationship.

One effective technique is the Swedish massage, characterized by long, flowing strokes and gentle kneading. This method promotes relaxation and helps alleviate muscle tension, making it ideal for couples seeking to unwind after a long day. Partners can take turns giving and receiving this type of massage, allowing each person to focus on the other's comfort and needs. By incorporating elements such as deep breathing and synchronized movements, couples can enhance their connection, making the experience not only therapeutic but also intimate.

Another technique to explore is the use of aromatherapy oils during the massage. Essential oils like jasmine, sandalwood, and ylang-ylang can elevate the experience by adding soothing scents that promote relaxation and emotional balance. Couples can create their own blend of oils and take turns applying them during the massage. This adds an interactive element to the practice, encouraging communication about preferences and creating an atmosphere of trust and exploration. The sensory experience of touch combined with aromatic scents can significantly deepen the emotional and physical connection between partners.

Hot stone massage is a more advanced technique that involves the use of heated stones placed on specific points of the body to relax muscles and improve circulation. Couples can learn to incorporate this technique into their routine by using smooth, heated stones or even alternatives like warm towels. The warmth from the stones can induce a deep sense of relaxation, making it easier for partners to let go of stress and tension. This technique requires coordination and teamwork, as one partner can focus on the placement of stones while the other enjoys the soothing sensations, fostering a sense of mutual care and support.

Lastly, couples should consider integrating mindfulness into their massage practice. Mindfulness involves being present in the moment and fully engaging with the experience of touch. By focusing on the sensations felt during the massage and the emotional responses that arise, partners can create a more profound connection. This practice encourages couples to communicate openly about their feelings and sensations during the massage, enhancing intimacy and understanding. By combining various techniques with mindfulness, couples can create a rich, holistic experience that nurtures both their physical and emotional well-being, paving the way for greater intimacy in their relationship.

Using Touch to Alleviate Stress

Touch has long been recognized as a powerful tool for fostering connection and intimacy between partners. In the context of alleviating stress, touch can serve as a vital means of communication that transcends words. When couples engage in intentional, loving touch, they create a safe space that promotes relaxation and emotional bonding. Simple gestures such as holding hands, hugging, or gentle caresses can activate the body's relaxation response, reducing cortisol levels and enhancing the overall sense of well-being. This physical connection not only alleviates stress but also reinforces the emotional ties that are essential for a healthy relationship.

Incorporating touch into a couple's routine can significantly enhance their yoga practice. Yoga itself promotes mindfulness and body awareness, which can be amplified through partner poses that require physical contact. These poses encourage couples to synchronize their movements and breaths, fostering a deeper sense of trust and cooperation. As partners engage in shared yoga practices, they can use touch to guide and support each other, enhancing their physical and emotional connection. This shared experience not only helps to alleviate stress but also cultivates a sense of unity and shared purpose within the relationship.

The impact of touch on stress relief is further magnified by the physiological responses it elicits. When partners touch, their bodies release oxytocin, often referred to as the "love hormone." This hormone plays a crucial role in social bonding and can lead to a decrease in heart rate and blood pressure, fostering a state of calm. Through consistent practice, couples can harness this biological response, turning everyday moments of touch into opportunities for stress reduction. Whether through yoga or other forms of physical connection, the act of touching serves as a reminder of the support and reassurance that partners provide to one another.

Engaging in touch as a means to alleviate stress can also enhance emotional communication. Couples who regularly practice touch are more likely to express their feelings and needs openly, creating a safe environment for vulnerability. This open dialogue is essential for resolving conflicts and deepening intimacy. As partners learn to communicate through touch, they may find themselves more attuned to each other's emotional states, allowing them to respond more effectively to each other's stressors. This increased emotional intelligence can lead to a more resilient partnership, capable of facing challenges together.

In conclusion, the integration of touch into a couple's life, particularly within the framework of yoga, offers significant benefits for stress alleviation. By embracing the power of touch, couples can enhance their emotional and physical connection, fostering a deeper sense of intimacy and partnership. As they navigate the complexities of life together, the practice of intentional touch can serve as a grounding force, promoting not only individual well-being but also a thriving relationship. By prioritizing touch and its healing properties, couples can create a nurturing environment that supports their journey together, ultimately leading to a more harmonious and fulfilling partnership.

CHAPTER 8: BUILDING EMOTIONAL INTIMACY

The Role of Vulnerability

The concept of vulnerability plays a pivotal role in the journey of intimacy for couples, particularly in the context of integrating touch with yoga. Vulnerability can be defined as the willingness to expose one's emotions, fears, and uncertainties. In a relationship, embracing vulnerability allows partners to connect on a deeper level, fostering trust and understanding. This openness is essential for building a solid foundation where both individuals feel safe to express their true selves without the fear of judgment.

In the practice of yoga, vulnerability manifests in both physical and emotional dimensions. As couples engage in yoga together, they often find themselves in poses that require not only physical strength but also the willingness to be open and receptive to each other's needs. For instance, partner poses necessitate communication and trust, as each partner must rely on the other for support. This physical interdependence can lead to a profound sense of vulnerability, where partners learn to trust each other's capabilities and intentions, enhancing their emotional bond.

Touch, when incorporated into yoga practice, significantly amplifies the experience of vulnerability. The simple act of holding hands, sharing a gentle embrace, or guiding each other through a stretch creates an environment where both partners can explore their limits. This tactile connection fosters a sense of safety, allowing couples to be more open about their feelings and experiences. The shared physicality of touch encourages a deeper exploration of intimacy, as partners learn to read each other's body language and respond to unspoken cues, creating a dynamic interplay of trust and affection.

Moreover, vulnerability can lead to personal growth within the relationship. By allowing themselves to be seen and heard, couples can confront their insecurities and fears together. This shared exploration of vulnerability can transform potential sources of conflict into opportunities for deeper connection and understanding. When partners support each other in navigating their vulnerabilities, they cultivate resilience, enabling them to face challenges as unified team. This growth not only strengthens their bond but also enhances their overall well-being, as they learn to embrace each other's imperfections.

Ultimately, the role of vulnerability in a couple's journey with touch and yoga is integral to nurturing a lasting relationship. By embracing vulnerability, couples can create a safe space where they can explore their emotions and deepen their connection. This journey requires courage and commitment, but the rewards are profound. As partners learn to navigate their vulnerabilities together, they cultivate a relationship built on trust, respect, and unconditional love, setting the stage for a fulfilling and harmonious union.

Exercises to Enhance Emotional Connection

Exercises to enhance emotional connection are essential for couples looking to deepen their bond and foster intimacy. As newlyweds embark on their journey together, integrating touch with yoga can create a nurturing environment where emotional and physical closeness thrive. These exercises can serve as a foundation for open communication, trust, and understanding, all vital components of a healthy relationship.

One effective exercise is the Partner Breathing Technique. This practice encourages couples to sit facing each other, close their eyes, and synchronize their breath. As one partner inhales, the other exhales, creating a rhythm that promotes a sense of unity. Holding hands can amplify this experience, as the physical touch reinforces the emotional connection. Over time, this exercise can help couples become more attuned to each other's physical and emotional states, fostering empathy and compassion.

Another valuable exercise is the Mutual Massage. This practice not only relaxes the body but also strengthens the emotional bond between partners. Couples can take turns giving each other a gentle massage, focusing on areas of tension or stress. The act of touching allows for a deeper connection, as partners communicate their needs and preferences. This exercise encourages mindfulness and presence, making it easier for couples to express their feelings and deepen their intimacy.

The Trust Fall exercise can further enhance emotional connection by building trust and vulnerability. One partner stands with their back to the other, who is ready to catch them. As the first partner falls backward, they must trust that their partner will be there to support them. This physical act can translate into emotional trust, as couples learn to rely on one another in a safe and supportive environment. Engaging in such exercises can help partners feel more secure in their relationship, allowing for deeper emotional exploration.

Lastly, the Heart-to-Heart Pose combines yoga with emotional connection. Couples can sit back-to-back, aligning their spines and taking deep breaths together. This pose encourages partners to feel each other's energy and presence while promoting relaxation and openness. As they breathe together, couples can share thoughts or feelings, enhancing vulnerability and intimacy. This exercise not only supports physical alignment but also fosters a profound emotional connection that can strengthen their relationship over time.

CHAPTER 9: NAVIGATING CHALLENGES TOGETHER

Common Relationship Challenges

Common relationship challenges can significantly impact the dynamics of a couple's partnership, especially for newlyweds who are still navigating the early stages of their union. One of the most prevalent issues is communication. Misunderstandings often arise from differing expectations and assumptions. Couples may find themselves in conflicts due to a lack of clarity in expressing their needs or feelings. In the context of integrating touch and yoga, open communication becomes essential. When partners learn to articulate their emotions and desires, they create a foundation for deeper intimacy and trust.

Another challenge couples often face is balancing individual needs with those of the relationship. Newlyweds may struggle to maintain their personal identities while forging a new life together. This balancing act can lead to feelings of resentment or neglect if one partner feels their personal space is being invaded or their interests are being sidelined. Through practices like yoga, couples can explore their individual journeys while also cultivating shared experiences. This dual focus on self and partnership can help maintain a healthy balance, allowing each person to thrive both independently and as a couple.

Additionally, couples may encounter issues related to physical intimacy, which can be influenced by stress, fatigue, or external pressures. The initial excitement of a new relationship can sometimes give way to routine, leading to decreased physical connection. This is where the integration of touch and yoga becomes particularly beneficial. Engaging in yoga together not only promotes physical closeness but also encourages couples to reconnect on a sensory level. Incorporating intentional touch during their yoga practice can enhance emotional bonding and bring awareness to each partner's physical and emotional needs.

Conflict resolution is another significant challenge that many couples face. Disagreements are natural in any relationship, but how couples navigate these disputes can determine the health of their partnership. Using touch as a tool for healing can transform conflict resolution. Simple gestures like holding hands or a gentle embrace during discussions can create a sense of safety and openness.

This physical connection can help couples stay grounded and focused on resolving issues rather than becoming entrenched in arguments. By integrating touch within their conflict resolution strategies, couples can foster a more harmonious environment.

Lastly, couples may struggle with external stressors that affect their relationship. Work pressures, family obligations, and financial concerns can create tension and distract from the intimacy that newlyweds seek to cultivate. Practicing yoga together offers a refuge from these external stresses, providing a shared space for relaxation and connection. It encourages couples to focus on their breath and physical presence, allowing them to momentarily set aside their worries. By acknowledging and addressing these common challenges through the lens of touch and yoga, couples can embark on a journey that not only strengthens their bond but also enhances their overall well-being.

Using Touch and Yoga to Overcome Obstacles

In the journey of intimacy, touch and yoga emerge as powerful tools to help couples navigate obstacles. These practices not only enhance physical connection but also foster emotional intimacy. When couples engage in touch and yoga together, they create a shared space of vulnerability and trust, allowing them to confront challenges more effectively. This subchapter explores how integrating these practices can aid couples in overcoming personal and relational hurdles.

Touch serves as a primary form of communication that transcends words. It can convey support, love, and understanding, particularly during difficult times. Simple gestures such as holding hands, hugging, or gentle caresses can significantly reduce stress and anxiety within a relationship. When couples intentionally incorporate touch into their daily routines, they build a stronger emotional connection, which in turn enables them to tackle obstacles with a united front. This nurturing aspect of touch can help couples feel more secure, allowing them to express their feelings openly and address issues that may hinder their relationship.

Yoga complements the benefits of touch by promoting mindfulness and self-awareness. Engaging in yoga together encourages couples to be present with one another, creating an opportunity for deeper connection. As partners move through poses, they learn to synchronize their breath and movements, cultivating a sense of harmony. This shared practice helps couples to align their energies, making it easier to confront challenges as a team. Through yoga, couples can also develop greater physical flexibility, which metaphorically translates to emotional flexibility, allowing them to adapt to life's demands more gracefully.

An essential aspect of using touch and yoga to overcome obstacles is the emphasis on communication. Couples should express their needs and boundaries during their practice. For example, one partner may prefer a lighter touch, or a specific type of yoga pose that feels more comfortable. By discussing these preferences openly, couples can create a safe environment where both partners feel respected and understood. This open dialogue not only enriches their yoga practice but also strengthens their overall relationship, providing a solid foundation for navigating challenges together.

Ultimately, integrating touch and yoga into a couple's routine can transform their approach to obstacles. By fostering a deeper connection through physical touch and mindful movement, couples can cultivate resilience and adaptability. As they face challenges hand in hand, they build a partnership grounded in trust and mutual support. This journey of intimate alignment not only enhances their relationship but also promotes overall well-being, allowing couples to thrive together in the face of adversity.

CHAPTER 10: CULTIVATING A DAILY PRACTICE

Designing Your Routine

Designing a routine that integrates touch and yoga can be a transformative experience for couples, especially for newlyweds embarking on a shared journey. By creating a structured approach to these practices, partners can deepen their connection, enhance their well-being, and establish a harmonious rhythm in their relationship. The key to a successful routine lies in intentionality, flexibility, and mutual understanding, allowing both partners to feel comfortable and engaged.

Begin by discussing your individual preferences and comfort levels regarding touch and yoga. This conversation is essential in establishing a foundation that respects each partner's boundaries and desires. Explore the types of touch that resonate with both of you, whether it be gentle caresses, supportive embraces, or playful interactions. Similarly, evaluate your familiarity with yoga practices. Some may prefer restorative yoga, while others might lean towards more vigorous styles. Understanding each partner's inclinations will help in crafting a routine that feels inclusive and enjoyable.

Once you have established your preferences, set aside specific times during the week to practice together. Consistency is crucial, as it creates a sense of commitment and anticipation. Choose a time when both partners are free from distractions and can fully engage in the experience. This might be early mornings to start the day with connection or evenings to unwind together. The environment also plays a significant role; consider a space that feels inviting and calming, adorned with soft lighting, comfortable mats, and perhaps soothing music to enhance the atmosphere.

Incorporate a variety of activities into your routine that blends touch and yoga seamlessly. For instance, you might begin with partner yoga poses that require cooperation and trust, fostering physical closeness. Follow this with a touch-based practice, such as massage or gentle strokes, which reinforces emotional bonds and promotes relaxation. Alternating between these activities allows both partners to experience the benefits of touch and movement, deepening their physical and emotional connection.

Finally, remain open to adapting your routine as needed. Life is dynamic, and couples may find that their needs and preferences evolve over time. Regularly check in with each other about what is working and what might need adjustment. This ongoing dialogue not only keeps the routine fresh and engaging but also strengthens communication skills within the relationship. By prioritizing this shared practice, couples can cultivate a deeper sense of intimacy and alignment, ultimately enriching their journey together through the powerful combination of touch and yoga.

Setting Goals as a Couple

Setting goals as a couple is a vital step in fostering intimacy and alignment in your relationship. When couples come together to establish shared objectives, they create a roadmap for their journey, enhancing communication and deepening their connection. By integrating these goals into practices like touch and yoga, couples can cultivate a harmonious environment where both partners feel supported and encouraged in their personal and mutual growth.

The first step in setting goals as a couple is to have open and honest discussions about individual desires and aspirations. It is essential for each partner to express what they want to achieve, whether those goals relate to health, career, or emotional well-being. By actively listening to each other, couples can identify common themes and areas of overlap. This process not only aligns their visions but also reinforces the importance of mutual respect and understanding, which are foundational elements in any relationship.

Once you have identified shared goals, the next step is to create specific, measurable, achievable, relevant, and time-bound (SMART) objectives. For example, if both partners wish to enhance their physical health, they might set a goal to practice yoga together three times a week. This not only promotes physical wellness but also provides an opportunity for touch and connection through partner yoga poses. By setting clear objectives, couples can track their progress and celebrate their achievements, reinforcing their commitment to each other.

Incorporating touch into the goal-setting process can enhance emotional intimacy. Couples might consider goals that involve physical affection, such as daily hugs or regular massages. These acts of touch can improve overall well-being and create a sense of safety and security within the relationship. Additionally, touch can be a powerful tool for communication, allowing partners to express their feelings and support one another through non-verbal means. As couples engage in their yoga practice, they can also explore how touch plays a role in their connection, further solidifying their bond.

Lastly, it is essential to revisit and reassess your goals regularly. Life is dynamic, and as circumstances change, so too may your aspirations. Setting aside time for these check-ins allows couples to discuss what is working, what isn't, and how they can adapt their goals to better fit their evolving relationship. This ongoing dialogue not only keeps couples aligned but also reinforces their commitment to personal and mutual growth, making the journey together even more fulfilling.

CHAPTER 11: CELEBRATING YOUR JOURNEY

Reflecting on Growth

Reflecting on growth is an essential aspect of nurturing a relationship, especially for couples embarking on a shared journey of intimacy and wellness through touch and yoga. As newlyweds, you may find yourselves in a unique position to explore not only the dynamics of your relationship but also the deeper connections that can be formed through physical and emotional engagement. This subchapter invites you to consider how your experiences with touch and yoga can serve as a foundation for personal and relational development.

Incorporating touch into your daily routine can significantly enhance your understanding of each other's needs and boundaries. Touch is a powerful form of communication that transcends words; it can express love, support, and reassurance. By engaging in practices such as partner yoga or synchronized breathing exercises, you allow yourselves to explore the nuances of physical connection. This exploration can lead to a more profound appreciation of each other, fostering an environment where both partners feel valued and understood.

Yoga, as a practice, is inherently reflective. It encourages individuals to tune into their bodies and recognize their emotions, which can be mirrored in a partnership. When couples practice yoga together, they not only strengthen their physical bodies but also develop a greater awareness of their emotional landscapes. This shared experience can open the door to candid conversations about growth, aspirations, and challenges, reinforcing the bond between partners. By reflecting on these experiences post-practice, couples can articulate their feelings and understand each other's perspectives more clearly.

As you reflect on your journey, consider the ways in which your practice of touch and yoga has transformed your relationship. Have you noticed shifts in how you communicate, resolve conflicts, or express affection? These changes often stem from increased awareness and intentionality in your interactions. By acknowledging and celebrating these growth milestones, you create a positive reinforcement loop that encourages further exploration and deepening of your connection.

Lastly, embracing growth means being open to change and the evolution of your relationship. As new challenges arise, whether they stem from personal struggles or external pressures, your practice of touch and yoga can serve as a stabilizing force. Regularly revisiting your intentions and experiences together can help you navigate these changes with grace. Reflecting on how far you've come and envisioning where you want to go can solidify your commitment to each other, ensuring that your relationship continues to flourish through every phase of life.

Continuing the Practice Beyond Yoga

Continuing the practice beyond yoga involves recognizing that the principles of yoga can extend into daily life, enriching relationships and enhancing overall well-being. For couples, integrating touch and mindful connection, as taught in yoga, can deepen intimacy and foster a stronger bond. This journey does not end with the completion of a yoga session; rather, it provides a foundation for ongoing connection through consistent practice and intentional engagement with one another.

One effective way to continue this practice is to incorporate touch into everyday interactions. Simple gestures such as holding hands, gentle caresses, or meaningful hugs can evoke feelings of closeness and security. These small acts of touch not only reinforce emotional connections but also contribute to physical health by reducing stress and promoting relaxation. By being intentional about touch, couples can create a nurturing environment that mirrors the serenity experienced during yoga sessions.

Another important aspect to consider is creating a shared space for relaxation and mindfulness at home. Designating an area for daily practice—whether it be for yoga, meditation, or simply spending quiet

time together—can enhance the couple's connection. This space should be inviting and free from distractions, allowing both partners to engage fully with one another. Incorporating elements such as calming scents, soft lighting, or soothing music can further enrich this experience, creating a sanctuary that encourages both physical and emotional intimacy.

Communication plays a vital role in continuing the practice of yoga beyond the mat. Couples should prioritize open dialogues about their feelings, needs, and boundaries. Discussing how touch and mindfulness practices affect their emotional states can lead to deeper understanding and empathy. By sharing experiences and thoughts, couples can explore new ways to connect and support each other's growth, ensuring that both partners feel valued and heard.

Finally, couples can explore activities that promote both touch and mindfulness outside of traditional yoga practices. Partner stretching, massage, or even dance can serve as avenues for connection, allowing couples to engage physically while deepening their emotional ties. By diversifying their approach to intimacy and connection, couples can keep their practice fresh and exciting, reinforcing the lessons learned through yoga and enhancing their relationship in meaningful ways.

CHAPTER 12: RESOURCES AND FURTHER READING

Recommended Books and Articles

In the pursuit of deeper connection and intimacy, couples can greatly benefit from a curated selection of books and articles that explore the integration of touch and yoga. One highly recommended book is "The Heart of Yoga: Developing a Personal Practice" by T.K.V. Desikachar. This book not only introduces the principles of yoga but also emphasizes the importance of personal practice, making it an excellent resource for couples looking to establish a shared routine. Desikachar's insights on deepening physical and emotional connections through breath and movement can serve as a guide for partners seeking to cultivate intimacy.

Another valuable resource is "The Art of Touch: A Guide to Sensual Massage" by David and Anna D. This book explores the therapeutic and sensual aspects of touch, providing practical techniques that couples can incorporate into their routines. It highlights the significance of mindful touch in fostering emotional bonds and enhancing physical intimacy. The authors provide step-by-step instructions along with illustrations, making it accessible for beginners. By integrating massage techniques with yoga practices, couples can create a holistic approach to nurturing their relationship.

For those interested in the scientific underpinnings of touch and its effects on health, "The Science of Touch: How It Affects Our Lives" by Dr. Tiffany Field presents compelling research. Dr. Field, a pioneer in the field of touch research, discusses how physical contact affects emotional well-being and stress reduction. This book is particularly beneficial for couples who want to understand the profound impact of touch on their relationship dynamics. The findings can encourage couples to prioritize physical affection, supporting their journey toward enhanced connection and intimacy.

In addition to books, numerous articles in reputable journals and websites offer insights into the integration of yoga and touch. For instance, "The Benefits of Yoga for Couples" published in the Journal of Couples Therapy discusses how shared yoga practice can improve communication, reduce conflicts, and enhance emotional intimacy. These articles often include practical tips for implementing yoga as a couple's activity, making it easier to engage with the material and apply it to everyday life.

Lastly, couples may find "The Healing Power of Touch" article series on wellness websites particularly enriching. These articles delve into various aspects of touch, including its role in healing trauma and fostering connection. By exploring these resources, couples can gain a comprehensive understanding of how integrating touch and yoga can lead to a more fulfilling and intimate relationship. The combination of scholarly research, practical techniques, and personal narratives can empower couples to embark on their journey toward intimacy with confidence and knowledge.

Online Communities and Workshops

Online communities and workshops have emerged as valuable resources for couples seeking to deepen their connection through the integration of touch and yoga. These platforms offer a unique opportunity for partners to explore practices that enhance intimacy and promote emotional well-being in a supportive environment. By participating in these virtual spaces, couples can engage with others who share similar interests and challenges, fostering a sense of belonging and encouragement as they navigate their journeys together.

Many online workshops focus on the principles of touch and its health benefits, providing couples with practical techniques to incorporate into their daily routines. These sessions often include guided exercises that promote physical connection, mindfulness, and relaxation. Couples can learn about the power of touch in enhancing communication and emotional intimacy, allowing them to express affection and support in new and meaningful ways. In these workshops, expert facilitators guide participants through various practices, ensuring that couples feel comfortable and confident as they explore the nuances of touch.

Online communities dedicated to couples practicing yoga and touch serve as platforms for shared experiences and collective learning. These forums allow members to exchange insights, ask questions, and offer support to one another. Couples can share their successes and challenges, creating a sense of camaraderie that can be incredibly motivating. Whether through social media groups, forums, or dedicated websites, these communities provide a wealth of resources, including articles, videos, and personal stories that can inspire couples to deepen their own practices at home.

The flexibility of online workshops allows couples to participate at their own pace and from the comfort of their own homes. This accessibility can be particularly beneficial for newlyweds who may be navigating the complexities of their new relationship while balancing work and other commitments. By engaging in these workshops together, couples can carve out intentional time for their relationship, prioritizing their emotional and physical connection. Additionally, the ability to revisit recorded sessions allows partners to reinforce their learning and practice whenever they choose.

Ultimately, the integration of touch with yoga through online communities and workshops can significantly enhance a couple's journey together. By embracing these resources, couples not only learn valuable techniques but also create a shared commitment to nurturing their relationship. The insights gained from participating in these virtual spaces can lead to healthier interactions, increased emotional intimacy, and a more profound understanding of one another, laying a strong foundation for a fulfilling partnership.

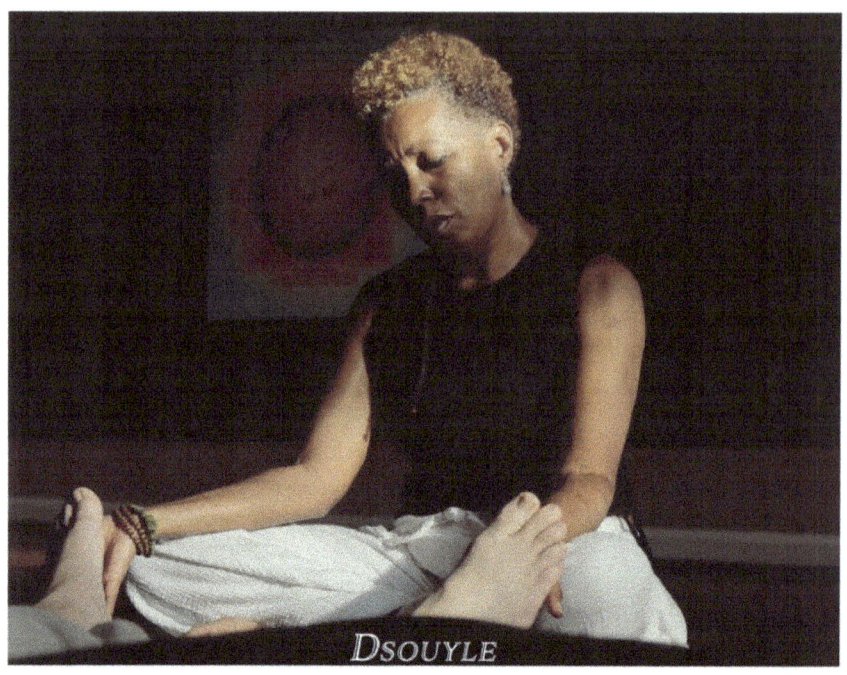

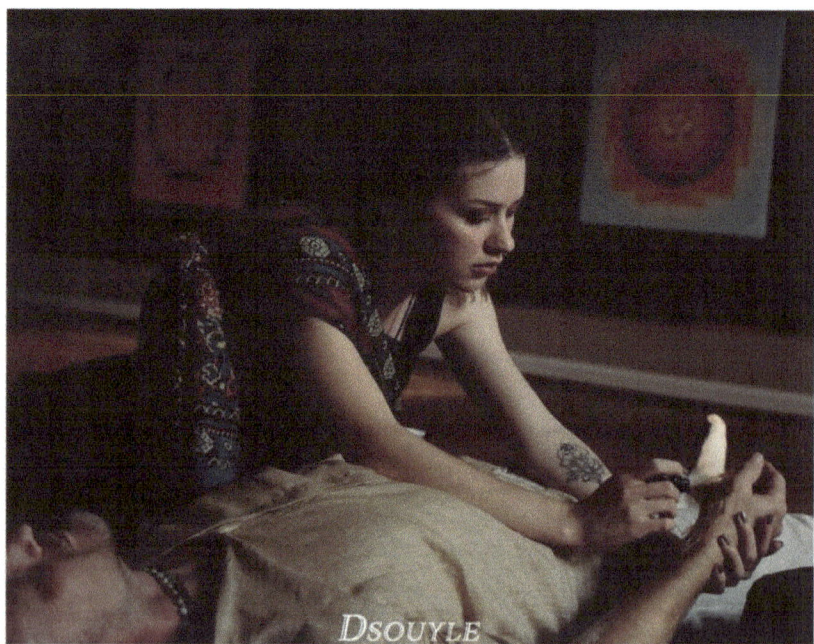

Intimate Alignment for Couples Through Touch and Yoga

Touch Me with Love

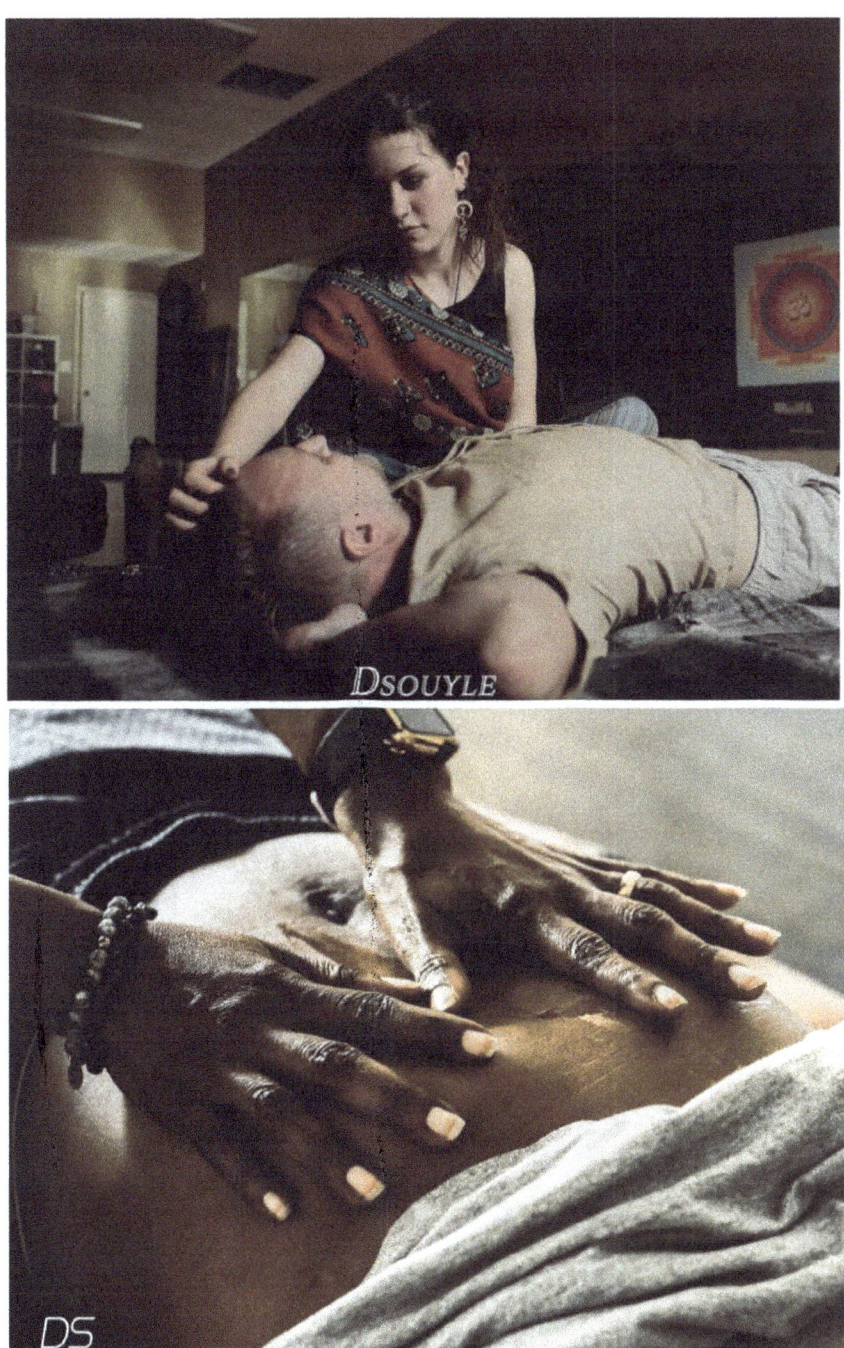

Intimate Alignment for Couples Through Touch and Yoga

Touch Me with Love

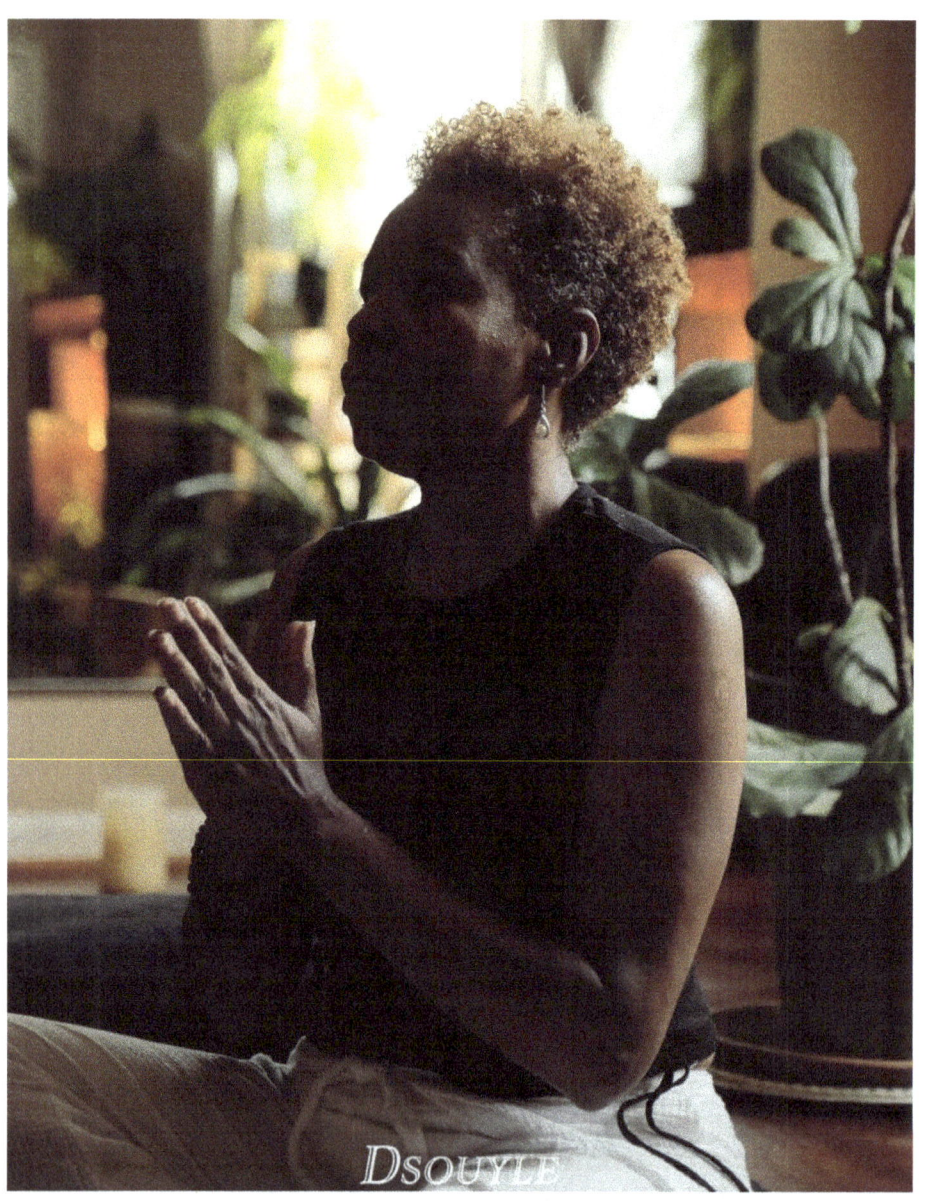

Enter The DSouyle Art Gallery

Intimate Alignment for Couples Through Touch and Yoga

CHAPTER 13: WELCOME TO THE ART OF TOUCH EXPERIENCE

Let's take a moment here and define a few words that will be used by your Certified Touch Artist who will guide you through the process of creating your own touch masterpiece with your hands.

Touch Deprivation is defined as experiencing the distress that arises from a lack of physical contact, which can manifest as poor, loveless, or inadequate interactions. This condition is frequently referred to as touch hunger or skin hunger, highlighting the deep human need for affectionate and meaningful touch.

Healing is defined as the gradual process of becoming sound, balanced, or healthy once again, restoring both physical and emotional well-being.

A Certified Touch Artist is someone who specializes in providing healthy, loving, and nurturing touch. In contrast to a massage therapist or other bodywork professionals, a Touch Artist focuses on guiding partners in igniting their imagination and establishing a sacred healing environment. This space allows them to let go of worldly concerns and connect intimately with Love, the all-encompassing everywhere evenly present force that binds all things together.

As we do in each of our classes, I welcome you to this healing experience with the Sanskrit greeting Namaste (which means I bow to the divine in you), and I invite you to make yourself comfortable. Today we will engage in an interactive experience that could change your life forever. I want you to get the most out of this sacred exchange so please turn off your phones and any other devices that may become a distraction.

Now, please sit upright in a comfortable seated position and breathe in and out slowly three times. We are in a sacred, safe space. Healing and restoration is our only aim. We welcome divine love as it fills this space and penetrates our hearts. And so, it is.

Continue to sit quietly with your eyes closed. As you continue to breathe, I want you to think back to the moment when you knew your partner was the one for you. If you are not with your intimate partner, begin to imagine the loving partner you want to attract. Hold that thought. Hang on to this feeling of bliss as you breathe in gratitude and exhale love. There is no limit to your access to divine love, so make sure you fully expand your lungs as you breathe in slowly and release with an audible sigh. Affirm to yourself silently (3 times), "My access to Divine Love is omnipotent, perfect, and always available."

Because we firmly affirm and deeply understand that divine love is truly limitless, we recognize that the love (which is so evident at the beginning of our relationships) never truly disappears or fades away.

Love can sometimes be obscured by the experiences that have caused us hurt or disappointment, but at any moment, we have the power to uncover that love and let it shine brightly through us, illuminating our hearts and the world around us.

Take one final deep breath in and let it out slowly, gently opening your eyes as you bring your awareness back into this room, back to this warm circle of light surrounding you. Please take a few moments to discuss what you just experienced, or write down your thoughts and reflections in your journal to capture the essence of this moment.

You are invited to be mindful and engage in self-reflection. This invitation stems from our belief that you are inherently perfect, whole, and complete as you are. We also recognize that you possess the remarkable ability to self-correct when any internal areas of imbalance or distortion are brought to your awareness, allowing you to align more closely with your true self.

Let's engage in a new exercise together. Extend your hands toward your partner and remember that any partner will do for this activity. Keeping a distance of one to two feet between you, close your eyes gently and focus your attention on any sensations you might feel in your hands. Now, take a step closer and once again, bring your awareness to the feelings in your hands. As you participate in this exercise, can you recognize how the energy within you and your partner connected despite the physical distance between your hands?

Finally, I invite you and your partner to find a comfortable seated position on your mat or the floor, ensuring that your backs are gently touching. As you take slow, deep breaths in and out, pay attention to the sensation of your back and your partner's back connecting, merging into one unified body. Sit up tall and straight, fully embracing the supportive presence of your partner behind you.

Intimate Alignment for Couples Through Touch and Yoga

Allow this connection to deepen with each breath, enhancing your sense of togetherness and stability.

Now I want you to take a deep breath in and gently lean forward as you exhale. As you continue this process, be mindful of your own comfort as well as the comfort of your partner. Together, breathe in and out three times, maintaining a steady rhythm. After this, slowly rise back up to a neutral position. At this point, allow your partner to take the lead. As they guide you, lean forward once more as you exhale. Focus on each other's comfort levels as you both inhale and exhale three times and then rise back up slowly to a neutral position once again.

If you both feel comfortable and safe supporting your partner's weight, now is the perfect moment to embark on a playful journey together. Allow your imagination to guide you as you maintain contact with each other's backs and begin to move in a gentle circular motion, first in one direction and then the other. Take a deep, calming breath in and fully exhale, releasing any tension. Now, return to a centered position. Each movement should be executed slowly, with the goal of harmonizing your breaths and movements with your partner. Closing your eyes and swaying to soft, rhythmic sounds can deeply enhance this shared experience.

In our retreats, attendees are introduced to a variety of partner yoga poses designed to help warm up their bodies, especially when the group mainly consists of singles. Remember, intimacy is not solely defined by sexual interactions. This experience teaches the art of touch as a nonverbal form of communication that speaks volumes of unspoken words while benefiting one's overall wellbeing. We want to break through barriers to intimacy, creating a space where we can freely love ourselves and extend that love to others.

Picture yourself in an expansive art gallery filled with studios showcasing works from various periods and genres. What mediums stand out you? Now, envision the artist's tools that transfer the images from their mind onto the canvas. In this session, hands, feet, and feathers are all instruments of creativity you may experiment with. We do advise against utilizing a bed for your artistic endeavors, as it may evoke connotations of sexual foreplay. Always remain mindful of your intentions.

Now, visualize an empty canvas resting on an easel in your art studio. How will you convey your expression of human creativity and imagination onto this canvas? Dr. Gary Chapman, the author of *The 5 Love Languages*, states, "Once you discover that physical touch is the primary love language of your spouse, you are limited only by your imagination on ways to express love."

You have set your intention and created a soothing atmosphere, correct? Now, with verbal or non-verbal consent to initiate touch, let us begin this journey. The Artist represents the giver, the one creating an artistic touch masterpiece from their imagination. The Canvas symbolizes the receiver, the individual allowing their body temple to be used to showcase a unique artistic expression of love. The Paint Brushes are the artist's hands, or any extensions thereof, which apply the artist's intentional thoughts onto the canvas. The Paint represents your massage oil or any other mutually enjoyable topical substance used to trace, sweep, glide, and stroke your canvas.

Who would you like to be first, the giver or the receiver? Take a moment to discuss this briefly with your partner. Another option could be for you to embody both roles, giving and receiving. In our live Art of Touch Classes and Retreats, participants have the opportunity to engage in solo practice, partner work, or one-on-one sessions with one of our Certified Touch Artists.

Are you ready to dive in? During live classes and retreats, we take the time to exfoliate one another's hands and feet. Then we moisturize them, ensuring they feel especially smooth. By layering sensory experiences, appealing to the senses of sight, smell, sound, and touch we add depth to our intimate moments together.

One of my personal favorite soundtracks for The Art of Touch Experience is "Song of Solomon" by the renowned jazz musician Ben Tankard. The instrumental pieces resonate with your soul, and the selections featuring vocals deliver romantic poetic prose. A fun and creative activity is to curate your own soundtrack using platforms like YouTube or Spotify. You can compile your favorite music into a playlist that is readily accessible whenever you wish to enhance this experience.

There are four essential movements that you will master as you embark on the journey to create your very own touch masterpieces.

Holding

Think of holding as a first contact on your blank canvas. Allow your intuition to guide you to the perfect place to softly place your brush(s). If you do not feel a gentle pull toward your canvas, try holding your hands 4-6 inches over each chakra (energy center), scanning for heat or other sensations. At any time, holding can be the primary artistic movement used in your masterpiece. When you decide to move your brushes on your canvas, consider creating lines or shapes like circles or hearts. Have fun with it as you explore the unique and hidden attributes of your canvas. You'll be amazed at what you discover. If your creativity is still not ignited, gently place your hands on the center of your partner's chest and hold. Breathe in and out slowly as you focus your intention on your partner's well-being and relaxation. Paint a colorful rainbow in your mind, through your body, now onto your canvas.

Tracing

Using your fingertips, trace along the brow and hair lines, and bony landmarks such as the chin (mandible) or collar bone (clavicle). Certain areas of the body/canvas require these specialized tools.

Focus your attention on how you feel as the artist while watching for facial expressions, sudden movements, or sounds that may imply discomfort. Our Touch Art Galleries boasts mutual satisfaction. With that said, be sure you are sitting, kneeling or standing in a comfortable position that does not cause you any discomfort.

Pulling

Fingers, toes, or other extremities can be gently pulled while creating your artistic masterpiece. Gentle hair pulls can also feel surprisingly stimulating. Try this movement as a self-care activity or with your partner. The more you are aware of what is truly enjoyable to you, the better you can effectively share it with your partner. Also, both men and women invest in hair extensions, so if you are not absolutely sure it's ok, do not insult your partner by pulling their extensions.

Creating art on your canvas by holding, tracing, and pulling can be so much fun, and if your partner has unique abilities or one or more of their extremities are no longer there, holding may be beneficial for soothing phantom pain. Amazingly, your desire to sweep away your partner's pain and your ability to be fully present can be an intimacy game changer in our rush-rush society.

Long Flowing Strokes

Continuous hands-on movement along your partner's legs, arms or back is what we call Long Flowing Strokes. Imagine wading water as you slowly glide your hands across the ocean. Speak peace to the ocean silently as the ripples turn into a complete calm.

Everything you see around you was created from a thought, and so it is with your partner. You did that. If you are familiar with Dr. Masaru Emoto's discovery of how our thoughts can change the molecular structure of water, then you can see the implications of how your thoughts affect your partner's body, which is composed of approximately 65% water.

Long Flowing Strokes, combined with thoughts of love, gratitude, peace, compassion, health, prosperity, and joy, seals the process of universal waters with the overtone tone of radiance. It's like magic.

Now that you have the essentials for creating your own touch masterpiece with your hands, take a few moments to reflect on your intention. Do you intend to attract your dream lover? Do you intend to soothe your partner and help them to release and relax? Maybe you and your partner have decided that your "at home" art of touch experience could be creative foreplay?

Remember, you and your partner are co-creating intimate experiences where you are both communicating in the language of love, so ignite your imagination. Feel free to create through the power of divine love.

What will you bring to your special experience? Consider a light, fluffy feather, your favorite nourishing natural oil, or maybe you want an edible aphrodisiac accompaniment. Think about it. You have a lifetime together to explore what makes you both feel good.

EnJoy your artistic journey together.

CHAPTER 14: MISCONCEPTIONS ABOUT TOUCH

- Touch is always a prelude to sex.
- Touching other people is not healthy.
- Children should be punished for touching in school.
- The majority of people who want to touch you have ill intentions.
- Therapeutic touch only takes place in a doctor's office.
- I'm fine without touch.
- The best place for touch is in privacy.
- Touching yourself is a sin.
- No one needs to learn how to touch.
- It's not a big deal if I choose not to touch others.

Thinking about misconceptions surrounding touch brings to mind the reactions I received after my very first interview concerning healthy touch for couples was published in The Detroit News over Valentine's Day weekend in 2006. The photo featured in this full-page story was quite similar to those in this book and was captured by a professional photographer in the newspaper's well-equipped photography studio.

Following the publication, the newspaper received a few complaints regarding what some individuals perceived as a lewd photo. In response to this backlash, the director of the massage school from which I graduated six years prior called me into her office for a discussion. During that meeting, she informed me that she was officially disassociating the institute from both me and my business venture, asserting that I was promoting an inappropriate link between sex and massage therapy, which she found unacceptable.

Ethical behavior as a massage therapy professional is absolutely non-negotiable and should always be upheld. However, when did the act of teaching couples how to share loving, nurturing touch with one another suddenly become deemed inappropriate or lewd? Most importantly, why didn't I ever receive an apology when the same school made the decision to add couples' massage classes to their curriculum? It is quite ironic that they had the nerve to label it "The Real Art of Touch," as if their approach was somehow more valid than mine.

Misconceptions often arise from limited or skewed perspectives that can cloud our understanding. If you hold the belief that touching is inherently negative, then reading this book may not be the most suitable choice for you at this time. However, consider that attending a live or virtual Art of Touch Experience might offer you a valuable opportunity to broaden your perspective. Engaging in firsthand experiences with loving, nurturing touch can unveil new insights and enhance your understanding of the subject. To truly benefit from this book, it is essential to approach it with an open mind and a willingness to consider a different perspective regarding how your body functions both individually and in connection with others.

In an insightful article about touch deprivation published in Massage Today, a respected trade publication, Ann Catlin, the founder of Center for Compassionate Touch, eloquently stated, "Our real work as massage therapists, regardless of your clientele, is to help usher in a new age where human touch returns to its rightful place in our world." This emphasizes the importance of touch in fostering connection and healing in our lives.

As far as I'm concerned, the rightful place for human touch is deeply embedded in our everyday lives. In the morning, when we rise and greet a new day, we should take a moment to embrace our body temple and affirm with conviction, "I love myself as a manifestation of God (Divine Love)." This affirmation resonates not only within us but also sets a tone for our interactions. When we greet one another, we should extend that same feeling of love and respect, recognizing that the person we are greeting is also a manifestation of Divine Love.

Throughout our day, there are countless opportunities to help usher in a new age where the warmth of human touch is prevalent and cherished. We are already connected through an invisible energy field that is active around the clock, continuously linking us. Touch serves as an intentional acknowledgment of this divine energy that flows through us all, bridging gaps and fostering deeper connections.

CHAPTER 15: APPROPRIATE & INAPPROPRIATE TOUCH

The news headline proclaimed, "School Enforces Strict No Touch Rules." In Fairfax County, Virginia, a school had suspended a student for simply touching another twelve-year-old child, sparking outrage among healthy touch advocates in both Michigan and Canada. The article noted that even a harmless high-five could lead to severe reprimands. In response to this troubling situation, we initiated an online petition aimed at Ending No Touch Rules in Schools to raise awareness about the absurdity of such policies.

The year was 2007, and now, as we step into 2025, the movement continues to gain momentum. Healthy Touch Awareness posters are being widely shared across various social media platforms, serving to educate the public about what constitutes appropriate and inappropriate touch. This initiative aims to foster a deeper understanding of healthy interactions for the betterment of humanity as a whole.

In the End No Touch Rules in Schools petition, one supporter from Missouri expressed their concerns: "Are we attempting to create robots devoid of emotions? Touching is an essential aspect of feeling. There are appropriate ways to touch and inappropriate ways, and this distinction must be learned through social interactions, especially in settings like schools. I strongly believe that we need to incorporate more lessons focused on morals, which should include guidance regarding appropriate forms of touching. How can we learn to shake hands or show camaraderie without physical contact?"

Another supporter from Michigan shared their thoughts: "Touch conveys so much meaning! My nephew, for instance, when he truly feels comfortable, safe, or loved by someone, will occasionally and ever so gently tap that person on the head. It represents his highest, purest expression of affection. I cannot fathom a world where he would be unable to express such a heartfelt endearment. My twin children, Josiah and Faith, both diagnosed with autism spectrum disorder and Sensory Integration Dysfunction, absolutely love to hug; they need these hugs, and they are eager to share their love with EVERYONE around them. The idea that anything could take this ability away from them is simply unfathomable.

The innocent, innate love that emanates from a child serves a very special purpose. It transcends all stereotypes and prejudices, reminding us of the fundamental connections we share as human beings."

A supporter in the Principality of Andorra wrote: "Nurturing children is so important. In a society where violence is prevalent in schools, the thought of no touch is ridiculous. We should educate our children on what's appropriate; not punish proper acts of caring for your fellow schoolmate."

In Pennsylvania, a supporter wrote: "Teaching in a kindergarten classroom, I would absolutely love to see this implemented! There is already so much sadness and distance in some children at this young age. A touch from a friend could mean so much."

A Connecticut supporter was enraged and wrote: "This is the most absurd thing I have ever seen. Touching is a part of friendship, love, and comfort. Kids who do not have a strong support system at home or have stress or problems should be able to comfort each other.

What kind of cold world do we live in where children cannot hug a friend, hold a hand or wipe a tear from a friend's cheek? Maybe if more children were able to comfort each other, they wouldn't feel so desperate for love and affection, maybe there would be less teen pregnancy, less violence, and more peace and much less feelings of craving the wrong kind of behavior.

Don't the schools know the saying Hugs not DRUGS. I think you have to be some cold-hearted jerks to even propose such an absurd thing. Wake UP people!! Kids need love and attention. Having a hug from a friend has gotten me through a rough day at school and in life in general. The power of touch is so vital to our lives. Imagine a world with no touching?

And who are the terrorists? I feel like America is losing its perspective on LAND OF THE FREE. Can't we concentrate more on what we can do to better educate our children instead of finding ways to strip our children of the right to be a kid and they wonder why kids bring guns and drugs to school. I hope sincerely that someone educates the EDUCATORS that are teaching children because they haven't a CLUE!!!"

The people voiced their concerns through the End No Touch Rules in Schools petition. In 2010, authors Sylvie Hetu and Mia Elmsater published a thought-provoking book titled "Touch in Schools: A Revolutionary Approach to Replace

Bullying with Respect and Reduce Violence." This impactful book presented the Massage in Schools Programme (MISP), which encourages children to massage one another, fostering a nurturing approach to health and well-being. The support garnered for MISP ultimately led to the establishment of the Massage in Schools Association (MISA), a non-profit organization dedicated to promoting this initiative in over 30 countries worldwide. This movement represents what I confidently refer to as a revolution.

In the aftermath of a global pandemic that has made social distancing and self-quarantining, often referred to as isolation, the new normal for countless individuals, will the people continue to speak out? Will the pervasive fear, combined with relentless media coverage of the dangers associated with physical touch—showing death and disease on television and the internet—continue to paralyze the American populace? An important question arises: will nations around the globe, which once thrived on regular expressions of loving touch in their everyday interactions, mirror America's anti-touch society, just as they have adopted the harmful aspects of the American fast-food culture?

There are many other powerful books that have been written over the past 25 years, which effectively illuminate the critical importance of healthy touch among both children and adults. Numerous experts consistently agree that a child's cognitive and social development can be significantly stunted when healthy touch is absent during crucial stages of growth, from infancy through to adolescence.

In our Healthy Touch Awareness 101 poster, we have introduced the concept of No Touch Zones as a more effective alternative to traditional No Touch Rules in schools. By clearly teaching this vital concept and ensuring its enforcement, we can create an environment where our youth have the opportunity to learn together, grow together, and interact with one another in meaningful ways. This approach imparts invaluable lessons about mutual respect for the human body and the essential principles of consent to touch, lessons that will carry over into their adult relationships, fostering healthier interactions throughout their lives.

In the midst of a global pandemic, where people everywhere sheltered in place, life as we knew it came to a standstill. Schools were closed, and the government, along with medical experts, urged us to self-quarantine to safeguard our health and prevent the spread of the life-threatening Coronavirus. Teachers, manufacturers, scientists, service providers, and entrepreneurs all found themselves masked and filled with a sense of fear and uncertainty.

"Keep 6 feet or more between you and others," they advised, while individuals grappled with the pervasive effects of the Winter Blues and Chronic Loneliness. This struggle was not limited to children; the elderly, too, endured profound suffering in silence. We witnessed on the news families performing drive-by visits, longing to see their parents and grandparents in senior homes, all while remaining in their moving cars, hoping to catch a fleeting glimpse of their loved ones.

Personally, I observed my father, who is living with dementia, diminish in both size and stature, a heartbreaking transformation fueled by the severe depression that stemmed from continuously absorbing the bleak news about #45's erratic behavior and the relentless COVID-19 death tracker that seemed to tick away hope. By March 2020, more than 282,000 lives had been tragically lost, according to the COVID Tracking Project, leaving an indelible mark on our collective consciousness.

At one point, my dad became absolutely convinced that he had contracted COVID and was on the brink of death. After hurriedly taking him to the hospital to confirm his fears, I instinctively turned to what I know best: the healing power of touch. I gently rubbed his neck, back, shoulders, arms, and feet, and miraculously, he seemed to come back to life. His overwhelming fear of the world spiraling into chaos and the haunting possibility of becoming just another statistic in the COVID death tracker weighed heavily on him, leaving him debilitated at times. I am profoundly grateful to God that I still have the ability to touch him and help soothe his pain during trying moments.

Let me be clear, though; I strictly adhered to all the COVID prevention guidelines because the last thing I would want is to bring home an uninvited guest who could potentially harm me or my dad. I also highly recommended that my clients take similar precautions, but I encouraged them to find creative ways, within those guidelines, to share the healing power of touch with their loved ones. I made sure to remind them that touch hunger, often overlooked, can also be a silent killer, affecting mental and emotional health in profound ways.

CHAPTER 16: TOUCH TRAUMA

Statistics have revealed that crimes involving inappropriate touch are often perpetrated by someone the victim knows personally. In my profession, I hear countless heart-wrenching stories that confirm this deeply disturbing and painful fact. My friend Dawn, who serves as a mentor for sexual and domestic violence survivors, shares her powerful testimony about how she found healing after enduring sexual abuse from the crib at the hands of her alcoholic father, a traumatic experience that shaped her life. Another poignant example is Dominique, a young lady I provided shelter for, who recounted how her own brother began fondling her and subsequently manipulated her into engaging in sexual acts when she was just 9 years old. The enduring trauma caused by such inappropriate touch can lead to severe mental illness and often results in devastating consequences, including homelessness, substance abuse, and even the tragic loss of life through suicide.

Atlanta Community Wellness Collective, a group I had the privilege of being a part of several years ago, hosted its inaugural Book Club gathering, where we chose the text "Angry Vagina" by Queen Afua to spark and enrich our monthly discussions. Our sacred circle consisted of women hailing from three distinct generations, with some traveling as far as four hours to participate in this important and divine appointment. It was truly remarkable to discover that 80% of the sisters in our circle, who were initially unaware of each other's experiences at the beginning of this journey, had each endured touch trauma. One by one, they bravely shared their deeply personal stories, shedding light on how their pain had been suppressed for many years, as they had previously believed they were the only ones grappling with such immense struggles. Their courageous openness fostered a powerful sense of connection and healing within our community.

Taking a moment to reflect on our seven basic chakras, we focus on the Solar Plexus, located in our upper abdominal region. This chakra represents our core self and our personal power. When it becomes blocked due to touch trauma, it can lead to physical, emotional, and psychological imbalances. Prolonged blockage of this chakra can result in chronic illnesses, digestive challenges, depression, and diminished self-esteem. The connection between our experiences and this energy center highlights the importance of healing and support within our circle.

To support the opening of your Solar Plexus, one could consider the idea of crowding out fast food and soda by consciously choosing to consume a greater variety of yellow foods such as squash, lemon, and ginger. Additionally, wearing the vibrant color yellow and incorporating yellow healing stones into touch artistry experiences can be immensely beneficial for your overall well-being and energy flow.

Personal accounts from numerous clients of mine reveal that childhood sexual trauma often acts as a gateway to various challenging behaviors, including self-mutilation, obesity, sensual fetishes, and even the re-presentation or projection of the perpetrator's behavior onto oneself or others. Imagine that for a moment. The deep pain and profound suffering caused by long-term childhood abuse can enslave you, transforming you into the servant of an invisible monster that lingers in the shadows of your mind and heart, dictating your actions and emotions.

Young women and men who suffer in silence and do not receive therapy or medical treatment often grow up to engage in relationships with minimal to no productive coping skills. They conceal their emotional scars and cry themselves to sleep at night, filled with fear about what might happen if anyone were to discover the trauma they endured during childhood. Despite their deep emotional pain, they hold onto hope, wishing and praying that they will find the perfect partner capable of loving them unconditionally, someone who can see beyond their struggles.

It is essential to recognize the profound impact of Post Traumatic Slave Syndrome (P.T.S.S.) on relationships within these communities. According to Dr. Joy DeGruy, an esteemed author and researcher, "P.T.S.S. is a theory that elucidates the origins of many of the adaptive survival behaviors prevalent in African American communities across the United States and the Diaspora. This condition arises from the multigenerational oppression faced by Africans and their descendants, a legacy of centuries spent in chattel slavery, a form of subjugation based on the erroneous belief that African Americans were inherently or genetically inferior to whites. This legacy was further compounded by institutionalized racism, which continues to inflict emotional and psychological injury." As the resident holistic health and life coach for an Atlanta community radio program, I had the enriching experience of hosting "Health & Healing

Chronicles" for several years. During this time, I had the distinct pleasure of interviewing an array of scholars and experts who specialize in various fields of health and healing. When asked about the significance of touch, they consistently Touch Research Institute at the University of Miami highlights numerous benefits of touch, including its positive impact on mental health issues such as depression and eating disorders, as well as its ability to boost self-esteem and even support immune function. Indeed, engaging in healthy touch practices can contribute to a robust immune system, which is essential for fighting off disease and maintaining overall well-being.

Recognizing that children often model their parents' behaviors and responses; it becomes imperative for parents who have experienced trauma to engage in healing practices that disrupt the cycle of trauma and other maladaptive behaviors. This is precisely why Certified Touch Artists are dedicated to holding space for divine healing to permeate the hearts and minds of participants in The Art of Touch Experience and Retreat. We collaborate with both local and national support organizations to ensure that we can assist our clients effectively, especially when their needs extend beyond our scope of practice. It is essential to understand that touch trauma should not have to lead individuals to a hospital bed or, even worse, to a state of despair. However, we know that timely and appropriate interventions have been proven to save lives and help individuals find their way to healing and recovery.

Let's take a moment here to pause and breathe in deeply, then exhale slowly. Now, let's affirm together three times, "My mind is purified through the power of divine love. I am healed." As you do this, visualize divine love surrounding you, cascading down like a shimmering foaming waterfall, enveloping you in its warm embrace. And so, it is.

Affirmations are definite statements or prayers that we intentionally feed our souls. Engaging in powerful affirmations, whether preceded or followed by a tone, chime, or vocal sound, serves as a significant pattern interrupter. This transformative practice, especially after an energy field clearing, can greatly support the channeling of positive energy and enhance mindfulness.

Now, imagine with me a world where touch hunger and loneliness no longer exist. Every human being is fully aware of the immense power within them to nourish and sustain themselves and their loved ones through meaningful and healthy connections with one another. This beautiful movement we are part of is actively healing not only the current generations but also the born and unborn generations to come. Is that a smile I see blossoming on your face? Can you envision our shared vision becoming a tangible reality? If you can see it in your mind's eye, take a moment to say to yourself, "loving touch can heal our world." Let this affirmation resonate within you as we work together to manifest this dream.

CHAPTER 17: YOU FEEL ME?

Google offered 3,900,000,000 results today when I searched the keyword "relationships." People everywhere are hungry for healthy, happy, loving relationships, and yet we find ourselves grappling with a pervasive sense of disconnection. Are we truly afraid to connect with one another on a deeper level? Have we come to accept a reality where it feels normal to walk past one another without even making eye contact, missing the opportunity for genuine connection?

A recent poll conducted among married men and women on the @optimallivingretreats Facebook and Twitter pages posed a poignant question: How do you feel when your spouse does not want to touch or connect with you intimately? The responses we received painted a vivid picture of emotional turmoil: "I feel rejected. I feel like he doesn't care about me. I feel angry and frustrated. I feel insecure in our relationship. I feel lonely, like I am yearning for affection. I feel foolish because I don't leave despite the pain. I feel unloved and unwanted. I feel like I want to end my marriage out of despair. I feel confused and lost. I feel needy for emotional support. I feel furious and resentful. I feel like I want to fight for what we once had."

In this intimacy alignment guide, you have been introduced to the transformative concept of touching with loving intention as a powerful means of enhancing intimacy in your loving relationships. You have been encouraged to actively crowd out feelings of hurt, trauma, judgment, and anger, replacing the empty spaces in your heart with forgiveness, love, joy, and peace. By doing so, you open the door to a deeper, more fulfilling connection with your partner, nurturing the bond that can lead to a thriving relationship.

"You feel me?" is a rhetorical question frequently posed by many participants during or after Art of Touch Experiences at retreats, churches, conferences, and yoga studios.

Here are a few of the testimonies that resonate deeply with attendees, showcasing their transformative journeys. "These are tears of joy! I have come to realize that

I don't have to leave this world without ever truly feeling alive in my body. I once believed my life was completely over. You feel me?" "I used to be afraid to touch my children because I worried that others would label me a pedophile. Now, I have gained a clearer understanding of what appropriate touch truly looks like. You feel me?" "I've been married for 30 years, and my wife hasn't touched me intimately in 10 of those years. I had no idea this was at the root of my anger and frustration. Do you feel me?"

CHAPTER 18: CONCLUSION

Hopefully, you will take away from this book that people's thoughts and feelings surrounding touch are deeply influenced by their past experiences and the knowledge we possess about our nature as human beings. Indeed, we do tend to shut down, construct walls, and lose ourselves in the misguided protection offered by external elements that do not deserve our trust, all while seeking refuge from those who wish to harm us. Yet, we also heal and learn to release the burdens we carry. We long to scream out loud, "DO YOU FEEL ME?" In response, we often hear an answer that resonates with our hearts, unspoken yet profound, "YES."

We truly live in this connection. It is important to understand that it is a privilege to receive the heartfelt request, "Touch me with Love." Such a request emerges from a space of genuine trust and vulnerability. Therefore, in the spirit of the foundational ethical principle of yoga, Ahimsa—do no harm—it is vital to consider the impact on the giver, who offers their entire essence as an artist. Allow them the creative freedom to express through the transformative power of divine Love.

Use your spiritual vision to look beyond the illusions of terror and despair that may permeate the atmosphere. Now is the time to activate the program that has been embedded in your DNA since the moment God declared, "Let there be light." Love and Light are the core of existence. Remember to express gratitude each day for the Son and the Spirit, who have guided you through the shadows and into the radiant light of Love. And so, it is.

The facts are indisputable. Every human being can greatly benefit from regular doses of raw, whole, nutrient-rich touch, infused with loving intention. Our seniors, in particular, deserve extra special attention and care. Grooming and personal care times present excellent opportunities to engage in touch that radiates love and affection. If you find yourself without a partner, remember to touch yourself. Your skin craves moisture, and your body thrives on your own touch each and every day. Drink plenty of water and take the time to touch yourself with love.

It is my heartfelt desire that this guide to intimacy alignment has resonated with your spirit, and that as you embark on the journey of creating your own unique touch masterpieces, you will tap into the wellspring of your creative genius. If you are not yet married and you are aware that your primary love language is physical contact, please consider this when choosing your spouse or partner. While it is certainly possible for anyone to become an artist in the later stages of their life, such transformations are not commonplace. Do you feel me?

I can't help but wonder: what if the question, "Do you feel me?" is the question of the century, echoing through our connections and experiences?

ABOUT THE AUTHOR

Versandra Kennebrew is a passionate motivational speaker, healing artist, and holistic health educator with over twenty years of transformative experience. Guided by her own powerful journey of overcoming homelessness and mental illness, Versandra has dedicated her life to empowering individuals, couples, and organizations to embrace optimal living, resilient thriving, and healing connections.

Known for her innovative approach to combating touch deprivation, Versandra has spent two decades teaching the art of touch—developing programs that enhance communication and intimacy among couples through techniques grounded in yoga, plant essences, and music. Her compassionate methodology fosters well-being and personal growth, encouraging others to live vibrantly despite life's toughest challenges.

Versandra's advocacy for social justice and poverty alleviation is deeply rooted in her lived experiences. She has served on prominent boards such as Health & Fitness ICU Detroit, the Coalition on Temporary Shelter Detroit, and Gateway Center Atlanta's continuum of care. As Community Service Commissioner for the Detroit Department of Human Services, her leadership has impacted countless lives. Through partnerships with the National Alliance to End Homelessness and the National Coalition for the Homeless, she continues to amplify the voices of marginalized communities and inspire positive change.

A natural leader and mentor, Versandra has coached hundreds of adults in personal development and self-care, while also mentoring elementary and high school students in leadership and communication. Her journey with Toastmasters International included recruiting and developing hundreds of volunteer leaders and facilitating club charters for 12 new clubs. She and her team presented over a hundred live and virtual leadership training sessions and retreats, which led to a substantial increase in Distinguished Toastmasters Clubs earning her the prestigious Program Quality Excellence Award.

Versandra has made her mark in broadcast media as co-host of Atlanta Radio's Health & Healing Chronicles and host of Optimal Living Starts Here on East Alabama's BEAM TV – a show dedicated to supporting military veterans and their families.

Intimate Alignment for Couples Through Touch and Yoga

An AmeriCorps VISTA alumna, recognized for her commitment to community and national service, Versandra remains dedicated to service both at home and abroad. She plans to further her mission as a Peace Corps Community Health

Facilitator while pursuing her Bachelor of Science degree in Exercise Physiology at Troy University. With credentials from Irene's Myomassology Institute, the Institute for Integrative Nutrition, and CYT-200 (certified yoga teacher), Versandra brings a wealth of expertise to her work. As the accomplished author of six self-help books—including Thank God for the Shelter: Memoirs of a Homeless Healer and her latest release Touch Me with Love: Intimate Alignment for Couples Through Touch and Yoga—she continues to inspire others to heal, reconnect, and thrive.

www.versandrakennebrew.com
www.youtube.com/@versandrakennebrew